UNSHACKLED MIND

# UNSHACKLED MIND

A doctor's story of trauma,
liberation & healing

CATHY WIELD

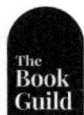

The
Book
Guild

First published in Great Britain in 2025 by
The Book Guild Ltd
Unit E2 Airfield Business Park,
Harrison Road, Market Harborough,
Leicestershire. LE16 7UL
Tel: 0116 2792299
www.bookguild.co.uk
Email: info@bookguild.co.uk
X: @bookguild

The manufacturer's authorised representative in the EU for product safety is Authorised Rep
Compliance Ltd,
71 Lower Baggot Street, Dublin D02 P593 Ireland (www.arccompliance.com)

This work is entirely fictitious and bears no resemblance to any persons living or dead.

Typeset in 11pt Minion Pro

Printed and bound by CPI Group (UK) Ltd, Croydon, CR0 4YY

ISBN 978 1835741 443

British Library Cataloguing in Publication Data.
A catalogue record for this book is available from the British Library.

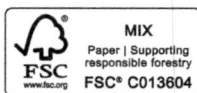

MIX
Paper | Supporting
responsible forestry
FSC
www.fsc.org    FSC® C013604

*For my family*

# Introduction

The purpose in writing this book is to illustrate the importance of a holistic approach when it comes to helping people to navigate the difficulties of an emotional crisis, whether it is short or more prolonged. I was myself caught up in decades of psychiatric treatment, which was based on a biomedical model, sometimes described as 'chemical imbalance'. I was also a survivor of considerable childhood 'adversity' which in my case was mainly attributable to being sent to boarding school at a young age. I was given a very poor prognosis and told I would never fully recover and I would need psychiatric drugs for life. There are others who may also believe that their situation is both hopeless and irreversible. It took years to discover the key to recovery, but at last I can genuinely say I am a thriving survivor of severe mental illness.

From time immemorial people have suffered with extreme emotional states. Whether this has manifested as incapacitating sadness or incomprehensible madness, the vast majority have recovered spontaneously when cared for by a loving community.

But institutional psychiatric care has had a dark history and there are many recorded accounts of people being imprisoned, tortured, and shackled to prevent their escape. Such overt cruelty has been abandoned in modern treatment of those deemed to be suffering from psychiatric conditions. But some have been diagnosed with serious or prolonged mental illness, and as a consequence are under chemical restraint as a result of high doses of psychiatric drugs. Furthermore, patients may be tied to the mental-health system, sometimes detained against their will and often with very little hope of recovery. I was shackled in this way until several lightbulb moments enabled me to overcome the negative prognostication given by very experienced doctors.

There are some potentially confusing terms used in this book which I will attempt to explain. However, trying to understand the use of drugs or 'medication' in psychiatry is a potential minefield. Drugs are chemicals which have effects on the body. When these effects are desirable, they are labelled 'therapeutic', when they are not helpful, they are labelled 'adverse effects' which is synonymous with side effects. There is no specificity when it comes to psychiatric drugs. A drug which alters serotonin levels in the brain, will also do so in the rest of the body regardless of which psychiatric diagnosis has been given. Many of these drugs have little variation in their chemical composition but are divided into various classes according to 'diagnosis'. For example, a drug that is classed as an 'antidepressant' or an 'antipsychotic' does not preclude their use in diagnoses other than depression or psychosis. This nomenclature has been derived from the marketing perspective of the pharmaceutical companies who need to make profits from their sales.

There are also many synonymous terms to describe what comes under the umbrella of mental illness. The passage of time, far from producing clarity, has further diversified the language in attempting to define what are essentially unique, personal experiences. There are degrees of suffering and degrees of self-identification as well as medically diagnosed, formal psychiatric disorders or conditions, all of which are interrelated. I cannot pretend to know the differences and therefore use descriptors such as 'mental-health conditions', 'mental illness', and 'psychiatric diagnoses' interchangeably to mean the same thing.

Language often seems grossly inadequate to describe unique emotional experiences such as anguish, sadness, loss, emptiness, fear, and hopelessness which when decontextualised and morphed into one become a generalised diagnosis such as depression. But I wonder if such labels do justice to those who suffer.

Yet it is important to recognise that there are some relevant similarities between individuals' experiences and people may find some consolation in knowing that others also feel the same way. But in order to be seen for who we really are, the context of our cultures, lives, and circumstances must be taken into consideration.

My first book, *Life After Darkness: a doctor's journey through severe depression* (describing what turned out to be only a transient return to a full and functioning life), was endorsed by the treating psychiatrists. We all thought that I had fully recovered from the seven-year nightmare as a psychiatric patient diagnosed with treatment-resistant depression, but it was far from over. There were many dark and difficult years when I was trapped, dependent on GPs, psychiatrists, psychiatric nurses, and therapists. During those periods of unrelenting and intolerable torment, I readily agreed to anything that might make me feel a bit better. But eventually the tide turned, and I started to recover, although it's fair to say that medical treatment did not provide the answers.

The decision to write this book has been a struggle, not just because it exposes parts of me I would rather keep hidden, but also because there are certain events I would rather bury and forget. I have changed my mind over what I believe, and this process has been long and arduous. I am reticent because I am compelled to be authentic; I have no wish to hurt or cause offence to the many good people who played their part and may not be comfortable with my changed perspectives. For this reason, I am mainly using pseudonyms throughout the book.

While I remain frustrated and/or disillusioned with certain systems and cultures still in place, it is not my desire to see individuals blamed or vilified. Those who cared for me professionally had the best of intentions whilst working under difficult circumstances. They did what they thought was right at the time.

Since the pandemic, many more people are looking for help with their mental health. Undoubtedly the pressures on society are immense whether as a result of poverty, no work or unsatisfying work, politics, discrimination, climate change, or just the frenetic pace of life; we must not ignore the societal factors which determine the health of every community. Regardless of the reasons for their struggles, no one should be stigmatised, and every individual deserves empathy, compassion and understanding alongside realistic practical solutions. This includes access to the right kind of support which will empower people to author their own turning. I suggest that, for many, the solutions will be primarily found outside of medical care. Here in the UK, we are lucky to have the NHS and many people expect to have their problems medically appraised. Unfortunately, long waits have costly implications which are more than just financial, while help is delayed for people in need.

There are recurrent themes throughout this book which may help you, your friend, or family member avoid some of the difficulties that I and my family faced, as a result of our ignorance and give you pointers to hasten recovery.

My own family were the secondary victims during the periods while I was a psychiatric patient. The medicalisation of my problems led to devastating consequences and robbed my children of any possible chance to lead happy, untroubled lives. Inevitably each one of us has our own unique memories of that time and in order to respect their privacy, I am writing only what is necessary for the narration of this story.

# PART 1

# Hurt not sick

# CHAPTER 1

# A place to start

It was the summer of 2017 and we had survived a shockingly turbulent year in Denver. I was much calmer and rather pleased with myself, despite the fact that I had weaned down my antidepressants, I had no symptoms indicative of relapse. However I was proactive and found a local counsellor, a psychotherapist, to help me process all that we had been through. A friend recommended Barb and I was lucky that she had an opening in her busy schedule.

## REFLECTIONS

On Saturday morning, I stood in the kitchen, chopping celery, mushrooms, and carrots to add to my version of lentil soup. The old-fashioned kitchen units were made from plywood and painted an off-white colour. There was a free-standing olive-coloured electric stove, and an enormous but ancient fridge freezer. I thought we might renovate sometime in the future when we could afford it, but right now it had to be low priority.

While I cooked, I listened to a podcast about the manifestations of childhood trauma in adults. My ears pricked up at the mention of a recording which coincidentally had also been referenced by Barb, my new therapist. Interrupting my culinary efforts, I spent a few minutes watching it on my phone. A baby was sitting in a highchair with her mother sat close by; she was watching her child, but her face was blank and expressionless. Apparently, this was part of a 'still face' experiment where the mother had been instructed to sit completely still and deliberately withhold normal reactions to her baby. At first, the baby was happy, gurgling away while the mother neither spoke, nor gave any signs of encouragement. But as the mother continued making no efforts to interact at all, the baby responded by becoming louder and more demonstrative. As this progressed, the baby became more and more frantic in her attempts to get her mother's attention until finally the baby's desperation erupted and she threw a tantrum, screaming, wailing, and throwing food from the highchair.

I quickly swiped my phone off and resumed the chopping, faster and harder. I felt such discomfort deep within my stomach as though I had witnessed some terrible ordeal. My little granddaughter threw tantrums occasionally and I had brought up four children; logically I knew it was normal to act out if they weren't getting enough attention. Then with a sudden intake of breath, I stopped. I was that baby. Then I laughed out loud, breaking the tension of such a ludicrous thought. But something clicked, and I thought more about the unpalatable theory that Barb had suggested to me on my first appointment.

## THERAPY

Sitting on a comfy blue armchair, I had tried to explain to Barb why I wanted counselling. "But", I said, "I don't need to go over the past." Clearly the years I had spent under psychiatric care had taught me nothing. Surely, I should have known that telling a therapist you didn't want to talk about something was a red rag to a bull. Barb wanted to know more.

Aged thirty-four, I visited my GP, convinced that recent circumstances, which included the triggering of memories of my childhood, were making me feel miserable. But this encounter marked the start of years of psychiatric drugs, ECT, and eventually brain surgery. The psychiatrists were convinced that I had a very 'biological, treatment-resistant depression' and, after my last hospital admission, I had been warned against psychotherapy that delved into the past, concerned that it might stir things up.

But Barb was obviously not going to be biased by the opinions of doctors on another continent, psychiatrists or not, and I found myself briefly outlining my life history. She looked startled, her eyes grew wider, and her jaw dropped as she asked me to clarify a few points.

"The symptoms coincided with Rachel's acceptance at ballet school?"

"Yes," I replied, "and I couldn't stop thinking about all my terrible memories of boarding school."

"And you were hospitalised on and off for a period of seven years?"

"But I made it home for almost all of the children's school holidays."

Barb shook her head as she dropped the bombshell.

"You were never depressed. You had PTSD."

I felt angry at her audacity. *Who does she think she is?* I thought. *She's not nearly as qualified as the extremely expert professors of psychiatry who know me so well and have treated me for over two decades.*

Barb had just poured cold water over their opinions, and I was paying her to do so. My gut reaction was to walk out but, shocked and unable to think straight, I agreed the date for the next appointment.

Once home, I had time to reflect. I kept Barb's opinions to myself, not ready to talk about it even with Peter, my husband of thirty-seven years. So here I was, stirring the soup, unable to shake her theory from my mind as I mulled over the implications of what she said, before finally deciding whether to cancel the second appointment. As a family, we had all suffered a great deal while I was a psychiatric patient. Could I really entertain the possibility that the diagnosis was mistaken when it had led to years of ghastly treatment?

## DOUBTS

The diagnosis of depression had changed my life and, even during the years of relative recovery, I was heavily invested in the psychiatric opinions regarding my illness. I had championed anti-stigma, written books and given talks about suffering with treatment-resistant depression. Undoubtedly, it made me more compassionate as a doctor, and I used my lived experience to educate colleagues about mental-health problems. But was I prepared to contemplate an alternative theory?

To date, no one else had validated what I had always considered to be significant and traumatic experiences of my childhood. If I had not been suffering with a biological illness, perhaps I was just weak. Perhaps I was to blame after all.

I remembered how awful it was to have my character pulled apart when some people judged me for not getting better. But the psychiatrists had always reassured me, telling me how ill I was. They said my brain chemistry was faulty and caused this endogenous or 'biological' form of depression. If Barb was right and I didn't have a brain disease, then where did all those symptoms come from?

The prospect of revisiting the past would be opening a can of worms. Yet I couldn't ignore my instinct as I had in the past, and the weird reaction to the podcast made me think there might just be something in what Barb said. This time, I owed it to myself to explore new possibilities. After all, Barb had confirmed my long-standing suspicion that nobody had really listened to what I was telling them all those years ago.

* * *

*It doesn't matter what background you come from, what role you play or what experiences you have had; you are the person who knows yourself best. Have you or someone you love been given a psychiatric diagnosis, which has left you wondering whether recovery is possible? Perhaps you have felt misunderstood or that your life story hasn't been heard. Perhaps you have wondered if your diagnosis is completely right. While the past cannot be undone, there is always hope for the future. While it took decades to unpick the truths about what happened to my younger self, that knowledge became part of my liberation.*

# CHAPTER 2

# Early life

When *Life After Darkness* was published in 2006, I wholeheartedly believed my psychiatrists' opinions, that my particularly severe case of depression was caused by a chemical imbalance and/or some faulty wiring in my brain. The details of my treatment during the period 1994 – 2001 are true, but I had accepted their interpretation of what happened. Now in 2017, if I was going to trust Barb, I would need to change my perspectives and face up to some very awkward questions, because the biomedical paradigm used to explain my depression had determined how the rest of my life unfolded.

## EMILY

In writing, I realise it is easier to describe myself as someone else. I have called her Emily. She has helped me retain some objectivity, as I examine the events of her life from childhood into adulthood which ultimately led a very muddled and vulnerable junior doctor to seek help from her GP back in 1994. Maybe I could become more compassionate towards her, rather than get on my high horse and judge her for her very obvious mistakes. Perhaps I can learn why she turned into the crazy, frenzied woman whose life was ruined alongside that of her family. Perhaps I may even commend her for the courage it took to survive and find it in my heart to forgive her.

It goes without saying that many children have problems growing up. But whatever their socio-economic circumstances, perhaps the greatest impact on children's future mental health is the relationships they have with the adult caregivers around them.

## INDIA

Emily was the second of four children born in India to a middle-class family. Neither of her British-born parents went to university but after the Second World War, George, her father, had taken the civil service exam and through a series of fortunate appointments, was able to enter the diplomatic service. Jane, Emily's mother, left school when she was sixteen, which was something she came to regret. She was very talented and intelligent with many interests and hobbies.

In India, Emily was looked after by an ayah named Poorna, until the family returned to England shortly after she turned two. Anticipating distress at the forthcoming separation, Emily's mother bought an Indian doll, dressed in a sari to console her. But Emily didn't like the doll, who was obviously a poor substitute for her beloved ayah. Although memories of India faded rapidly, whenever Emily came across the doll, more often than not in the back of a cupboard, it prompted her to ask about Poorna.

## KENYA

The family moved to Nairobi and at age four, Emily started school in the kindergarten class of the Loretto Convent. Despite the family's lack of religious affiliations, Emily took easily to the Catholic ritual; she liked going to chapel, dabbing her forehead with holy water and curtseying before the altar, mesmerised by the crucifix which was also depicted in the stained-glass window high above. Her mother relates with amusement how one day Emily came home saying she had seen God: "They keep him in a box". But when she requested a white dress to have "tea with Jesus", her parents realised it was a little more serious. Emily, along with the rest of her class, were being prepared for first communion and she had not been baptised into any church, let alone as a Catholic. Naturally it was very confusing as Emily was far too young to understand why she was suddenly prohibited from going to chapel and relegated to the Protestant class instead. It seemed quite normal when children were reprimanded for their misdemeanours, which at times resulted in being rapped across the knuckles or struck on the back of the legs. But it was different the day Emily found herself being shaken by the shoulders for daydreaming. It was bewildering the way grown-ups suddenly flared up.

## PUZZLED

Before they left India, Emily had been at death's door, seriously ill with complications of measles. Now in Kenya at age six, she was hospitalised for a second time. In those days parents were not allowed to stay with their sick children and Emily was very frightened, isolated in a room all by herself with severe gastro-enteritis. She could hear a nurse shouting at one of her young patients, "Stop that coughing, Bronwyn."

It was a relief to get back home to her family and their pets in the single-storey bungalow surrounded by so many colourful bushes and trees. They had a black-and-white cat called Frankie, who gave birth to kittens in the toy cupboard, and two dogs – a boxer and a dachshund. Emily and her older brother, Andrew, fed a hedgehog trapped in the walled rockery garden, named Stinker, for obvious reasons. She loved the way Jane, her mother, called them over to take a look at a chameleon or perhaps a praying mantis sitting on her finger. The garden was beautiful. There was bougainvillea covered in purple flowers, jacaranda, a tall avocado tree, as well as paw-paws, banana trees and passion fruit. Emily's parents installed a climbing frame, and she spent many a happy hour clambering around and hanging upside down from precariously high positions.

At weekends the family often went on excursions that today would be seen as luxury holiday events. They went to the game parks and Emily experienced both the thrill and the anxiety while they drove closer to get a good view of the rhinos. Spotting elephants, giraffes, lions, and other big cats was much more relaxing. They made trips to Lake Naivasha with its very distinctive fishy smell and its large flocks of pink flamingos and Emily has fond memories of walking the dog with her father, taking paths through fields where the maize grew taller than she was. The family never had television while they lived overseas but sitting on the back seat of the car next to her brother, watching the big screen at the drive-in cinema was a treat. This was Emily's normal home life; she knew no different.

It was probably as a seven-year-old that Emily first became conscious that her skin wasn't black like the Africans. Emily spoke Swahili and often visited the servants' quarters – a separate small building consisting of a couple of rooms, set back from the main house. Henry the cook was always such fun, with his big flashing smile. Emily squatted down on her heels, watching, while they pounded mealie into flour, and she savoured the smoky smell as it cooked on a charcoal burner to make Ugali. Although she didn't understand why their home was so different to her own, she still regarded herself as part of their family. Until one day, for no apparent reason, she was no longer welcome.

## SURPRISES

Always imaginative, Emily had an idea: she told her friend Melanie that she wanted to become an African, and off they went to the fishpond, where they covered themselves in mud. Proud of herself, Emily went to show Jane what she had done. "Look at me, I'm an African."

Jane was heavily pregnant, and engrossed in a book as she sat in the warm sunshine. She didn't look up until Emily's voice became insistent. Then she shot up from her chair and took the two little girls by their arms, and quickly scuttled them into the house, straight to the bathroom, where she hosed them down. Emily couldn't understand what she'd done wrong.

When Jane went to the hospital to have the baby, George drove the children down the long, dusty, orange murram road to Mombasa. They always loved going to stay at the small, thatched bungalow on the beach, which was used by High Commission families for R&R. But poor Emily suffered with frequent styes, and on this occasion she became very unwell as the infection spread until one side of her face became red and swollen. Despite George's best efforts to cheer her up, even the new swimsuit with a little skirt attached didn't help, they were forced to make an early return to Nairobi so Emily could receive hospital treatment. But all was soon forgotten when they arrived home to the most wonderful surprise – a new baby sister.

## FUTURES

The children adapted easily to their frequent moves; the stability was in the family, rather than a consistent locality. But a perk of working overseas for the Foreign Office was that the government funded the payment of boarding school fees alongside the travel costs for two school holidays per year. British diplomats were expected to send their children back to the UK for their education by the time they reached secondary school age, if not before.

This was not the accepted practice for most other nationalities in similar positions and there were usually English-speaking international schools of some description in most larger towns and cities where Foreign Office missions were located. Under normal circumstances George and Jane would not have been able to afford the fees and as the children grew up, they were repeatedly reminded of the privilege they would have in being sent to boarding school.

It was just weeks after Sonia's birth that the family drove to the airport to see eleven-year-old Andrew off for his first term at boarding school. They stood together on the viewing platform above the terminal and watched him walk across the tarmac, dressed in his new school uniform; he paused briefly to turn and wave, before ascending the metal stairway to board the plane. Emily was blissfully ignorant of what this 'privilege' meant for him, or for her own future either.

## VOYAGE

The Kenya posting came to an end that September and the family minus Andrew returned to England by sea. On board the ship, Emily was thrilled to be enlisted as mother's little helper. When the ship listed from side to side, she passed Jane what was needed to change her adorable baby sister's nappy. Emily loved pulling faces and tickling her tummy as Sonia mastered the art of smiling.

The closure of the Suez Canal prolonged the voyage as they had to sail around the Cape Horn, which was no hardship for any of the child passengers who entertained themselves. There was only one shop on board the passenger liner and Emily stared longingly at a doll in the window. Her parents bought 'Heidi' for her eighth birthday. Emily was indeed privileged, part of a family who loved her, and was leading an extraordinarily rich and varied life. No wonder George and Jane kept reminding their children just how lucky they were.

## IMAGINATION

Back in England, George was delighted by the news of his next posting to Chiang Mai in Thailand where he would be the British Consul. It was considered to be one of the most idyllic jobs that a diplomat could wish for. But first George had to attend Thai language training at the School of Oriental and African Studies, in London. Jane stayed at home caring for her two little sisters and Emily was enrolled at the local primary school. In the spring, Great-Aunt Elizabeth came to stay. A widow, without any children of her own, she was soon besotted with baby Sonia and Emily felt usurped from her prime position as mother's little helper.

It was only half a mile to school and Emily happily walked this on her own. One morning during assembly, the headmaster issued a warning that children should not talk to strangers. By the afternoon walk home, Emily, who was particularly good at writing stories, had incorporated this into one of her tales. When her mother made the usual enquiries about her day, she told her that a man had stopped her on the way to school and demanded sixpence to let her go past. Great-Aunt Elizabeth was listening and saw through it straight away, but Jane was alarmed and immediately came to her defence. "Emily would never tell such a lie."

Now Emily found herself unwittingly caught in the conflict between her mother and her great-aunt. Of course, her aunt was right, but away from Jane's watchful eye, she was often unkind to both Emily and her little sister, Margaret. The look in Great-Aunt Elizabeth's eyes froze Emily to the core and she didn't know how to back down. Meanwhile Jane called the police.

Two uniformed policemen called at the door and the

petrified Emily was shepherded into the dining room, where they all sat round the oval rosewood table. Emily knew that bad people were taken away and put in prison and if they found out she was lying, she knew that was exactly what was going to happen to her. One of the policemen took out his notebook and she described her fictional man and furnished the police with details of what she thought might have happened. The more questions they asked, the further she embellished the story. But it didn't end there. On her own in the back of the police car, she was driven around the neighbourhood in search of the alleged extortionist.

When bedtime finally came, Emily lay on the top bunk crying quietly, trying not to wake Margaret who slept soundly on the bunk below. During the preceding few weeks, Emily knew she had been very naughty; she had stolen a lollypop from the sweetie shop and several times she had helped herself to a couple of silver coins which George had left on his dressing table. One day, Jane had asked if she knew what had happened to half a crown that had gone missing from her purse. In fact, Emily had become quite adept at supplementing her pocket money to buy sweets which she generously shared with her friends. But as she lay there that night, Emily had an epiphany; suddenly she realised how wicked she had been, and her conscience was stricken. Only now it was so much worse because if the police found out, she would be sent to jail. Not knowing how to put it right, Emily cried and cried until finally she fell asleep.

The next day brought no respite. Surely Great-Aunt Elizabeth knew everything, and Emily was a naughty, fibbing, good-for-nothing child. By now, she was far too scared to confess to either of her parents and there was nobody else to reassure her or correct her childish fantasies. The police drove Emily to school and picked her up for the next few days, all the while searching for a man who didn't exist, who had not threatened her or demanded anything from her. It almost fooled Emily into thinking her story was real. But the police were losing patience.

One day, they stopped the car at the side of the road; there was a slight incline, and the trees were in leaf, overshadowing the pavement. It fitted Emily's sinister imaginings as the place where the incident had occurred. The police were eager to know where the man had gone from there – in desperation Emily pointed to a tall wooden gate in a fence, behind which appeared to be a forested area – of course, she had no idea what was behind it. They left her by herself in the car and went inside. She was surprised when they came out shaking their heads. She was expecting them to emerge with the culprit, hands cuffed behind his back. "No, he didn't go in there", they said. They took her back home and that was that.

Maybe the police closed the case, but for eight-year-old Emily, it was far from over. Her parents had no idea what was going on in their little girl's mind as she tried hard to atone for her wrongdoings and that meant she tried to be very, very, well behaved. It was the sixties, when many parents at that time were not demonstrably affectionate, neither were children's feelings a topic of discussion. Emily's parents were no exception; they were quick to correct or reproach their children but gave little in the way of approval or affirmation. Even so, Jane often commented on what a sensitive child Emily was. Every time Emily was told off, she took it to heart, as she remembered what a bad girl she was.

## INSIGHT

The family travelled to Venice to board a ship headed for Bangkok, and Emily finally found welcome reprieve. At last, she felt safe from the reach of the police, although her guilty feelings were never far from the surface.

When Emily crossed the threshold in understanding the

difference between right and wrong, it should have been for her greater good. Her physical needs were provided for, yet shortly after the birth of her baby sister she had developed a predilection to lie, cheat and steal. When Great-Aunt Elizabeth came to stay, she doted on baby Sonia to the expense of both Emily and four-year-old Margaret. Presumably Jane was preoccupied with her two youngest children and the forthcoming move, while George was busy learning a new and difficult language. Perhaps in the mêlée, Emily was just trying to get her emotional needs met and perhaps the recent onset of bad behaviour was a subconscious attempt to get her parents' attention. But it backfired and Emily became convinced she was wicked.

Photos up to this time show a little girl with a cheeky grin. But afterwards, Emily lost her confidence and with it, her sunny nature. Her furtive imagination was her downfall and the consequences were life-changing as she absorbed inaccurate and immature beliefs about her self-worth into her developing personality.

The middle classes were a stiff-upper-lip society, and children were expected to be obedient and well behaved, rather than mollycoddled with too much love or affection. George in particular was keen that his children learn to be independent and stand up for themselves.

So, the foundation was laid for Emily to accept a fundamentalist view of Christianity. As a teenager, she needed no persuasion to believe that she was born a sinner, deserving punishment, nor that without God to rescue her, she was doomed to suffer eternal damnation.

Once she turned to Christianity, Emily repeatedly asked God for forgiveness and even as an adult, if complimented Emily felt an imposter, but had no difficulty in believing that others were good. Somewhere deep inside, the young child Emily lived on, prone to feeling guilt for even trivial and minor infractions of her strict moral code, and unable to believe that she was truly loveable.

## AT SEA

Air travel was becoming more and more affordable, so the voyage to Thailand was the last time the family travelled by sea. Maths and English workbooks kept Emily occupied for an hour at most, and then she was free to go and play with the other children who were on board the ship. The crew were very tolerant of the kids, as they explored below deck, even venturing into the engine room. At other times they could be found leaning over the railings watching the high waves and rolling seas or counting the flying fish. Storms provided additional excitement, while they were sprayed by the angry waves, and then inside they roamed the passageways, laughing as they tried to keep their balance while the ship listed from side to side.

When the ship crossed the equator, there was a special party for everyone on board. Emily was both mesmerised and horrified as the crew enacted a mock operation, pulling sausages from the 'patient', accompanied by a liberal amount of tomato sauce, before hurling him into the swimming pool. During the remaining weeks at sea, the children spent most of their time playing in and around the pool in the sunshine. Emily hadn't forgotten her terrible ordeal back in England, but at least it had retreated to the back of her mind.

## BANGKOK

Bangkok was hot and humid, a busy, noisy city but the family soon settled into their new life. George still had some further language training to complete before they moved north to the consulate in Chiang Mai. Emily and Margaret were enrolled at the local British primary school, smart in their new, green gingham uniforms. The buildings that housed the classrooms were Thai style, on stilts, raised above ground due to the perennial risk of flooding during monsoon season. School hours were 7am until 1pm to make the most of the cooler part of the day as little air moved through the open windows. The curriculum was typical for a primary school, but with the addition of Thai language lessons. Emily found little difficulty in picking up a new language and soon became friends with one of her Thai neighbours. They took her to traditional Thai dance classes, but she much preferred her ballet lessons. When the dance school became involved in a performance of *Sleeping Beauty*, Emily's ballet teacher was the Lilac Fairy. Emily was cast as a snowflake and her father photographed her on the steps of the theatre, proudly wearing her tutu.

One day without any warning or preparation, Emily was summoned to the school office to sit an entrance exam for boarding school. It didn't worry her because she was an avid reader and loved the *Chalet School* series which portrayed boarding school to be full of fun and adventure. However, Emily did ask her mother if she could go to a ballet school instead, but such unrealistic notions were soon dispelled from her mind.

How trusting these parents were, to send their children thousands of miles away to a school where they would be looked after by strangers they had never met. Yet Emily's parents prohibited her from watching the movie *Oliver!* because they thought she was too sensitive, and it might give her nightmares.

George was due some leave before they moved to Chiang Mai. It was the perfect opportunity to kit Emily out, ready for her first term at boarding school. She was reminded how lucky she was to have the privilege of a public-school education.

\* \* \*

*Whatever their backgrounds children are at the mercy of adult caregivers, especially when they spend a large proportion of their lives away from loving homes. They remain vulnerable even if they are removed for their own protection and are at risk of abuse or neglect. They may not receive enough 'parental' love and care. What was your experience when growing up? Do you think your emotional needs were met?*

# CHAPTER 3

# Boarding school

I wonder what motivated the writers of children's fiction to make the idea of boarding school sound such fun. Although boarding school may provide respite for some unfortunate children who have a difficult home life, for very many children it is the complete opposite.

## FIRST DAY

The first day at school is a sentinel event which becomes firmly fixed, separating life into before, and after. Often it is remembered in a similar way to the experiences of profound shock or sudden loss. Memories may be completely absent or surprisingly lacking in detail around a day that changes that child's life forever, or alternatively the memory is preserved, intense and vivid.

Emily cannot remember what day she left home or who was with her when they drove to Bristol. She has no memory of the drive through the gates, into the walled grounds with the playing fields on her right, that later seemed so big. She cannot remember arriving or their car being parked in the small, empty playground with a seesaw and a couple of swings. Neither does she remember going up the stone steps or through the double doors into the junior school building. She only remembers the smell of the place, the mixture of aromas created by floor polish and pine disinfectant.

Her trunk must have been taken out of the car and it's likely that her parents came upstairs with her to the dormitory. She cannot remember saying goodbye or the moment they left, but she vividly remembers standing by her bed feeling as though she had been knocked over by a large wave. She couldn't breathe, as if underwater with a mixture of sand and sea in her mouth and nostrils, being rolled over and over again. When she finally came up for air, she found herself bereft, abandoned and totally alone.

With this came the sudden insight that boarding school was not going to be anything like the books she had read. It must all be a terrible mistake and she wanted Mummy and Daddy. But they had left her behind, all by herself and she felt betrayed. She doesn't remember crying, she only remembers being shouted at to stop. She soon learned that tears must only be shed silently, secretly, under the sheets at night.

There were seven beds in the dormitory, three down one wall, four down the other, all identical with narrow iron bed-frames evidently painted white some time ago. The girls had to make up their own beds, using 'hospital corners' for neatness. There was a wooden chair beside each bed and space for their clothes was allocated to specified drawers in the chests located beneath the windows. But before anything could be put away, all items had to be neatly folded on the bed for the inspection by the matrons. Anything not specified on the uniform list was not allowed and, once confiscated, was never seen again. The girls became adept at secreting away torches, sweets, or other forbidden items. Miss Sourpuss and Miss Meany were the matrons in charge of the little girls' welfare in the junior school and they made no attempt to show concern or offer comfort. Even though Emily had lived in many different places, nothing about this bore any resemblance to home. She was lost. On that very first night, Emily the new girl was quizzed, "Do you know where babies come from?"

Seeing her hesitation, the other girls gathered round, and she was initiated with an impromptu lesson on sex, puberty, and periods. Any residual notions that school was going to be fun left, along with her innocence. It might have seemed that Emily was suddenly forced to grow up, but the truth was that her nine-year-old self was forced into hiding.

## DORM LIFE

The dormitory (dorm) was a microcosm of school life where the girls spent hours together unsupervised. The matrons appeared vigilant, well able to spot anyone who broke the rules, yet they seemed blind to the bullying; in the dorm there was no escape and nowhere to hide.

How ironic that only a year earlier Emily had been terrified of being sent to jail and here she was, in a sanctioned prison for children of privilege, funded by the state. Every aspect of the girls' lives was regulated by the timetable, and they had no control over what they did, when or where they did it. Thrown together devoid of the presence of loving and supportive caregivers, the girls found their own way to survive and, for many, it cost them dearly. Showing emotion was strongly discouraged, and the new girls took the lead from those who had been there longer. They were soon indoctrinated to believe that it was weak to admit to unhappiness or homesickness, so the children became pros at internalising and suppressing their feelings. They didn't know that their peers also felt miserable or lonely, so it was easy to feel isolated surrounded by the fallacy that the other girls were happy.

Emily certainly saw it that way. She thought the other girls, even her friends, didn't really mind being at school. Thinking they were strong in the way they coped, her beliefs about herself morphed – not only was she bad, she was also weak as well. It was only as an adult, reading about this unique boarding school phenomenon and talking to some school friends, that I discovered they felt much the same way as she did. But such insights came far too late for nine-year-old Emily.

## RESPONSIBILITIES

Emily didn't blame her parents. She knew Foreign Office children were expected to go to boarding school. As the first generation in the family to be sent away to school, her parents had no idea that there could possibly be any downsides. They believed the fantasy that boarding school would be the children's best days of their lives and they believed it would enhance their chances to go to university, and open doors to further opportunities later in life. They were grateful for their good fortune and thought Emily should be too.

Of course, some children apparently thrive at boarding school, but Emily was not one of them. She had a happy home life and the disparity between expectation and reality was not just confusing, it was agonising. She hated going away, she hated school, and she was too young to articulate her feelings. Not only did she feel abandoned, it felt like punishment. Her parents could not see what was going on in her world and she couldn't fight their logic. Her father meant well when he laughed at her complaints. His favourite response was, "It will do you good, toughen you up."

Having already perfected her ability to blame herself, the more Emily heard that school was good for her, the more isolated and shut down she became. Without the comfort she craved, she had little chance of learning healthy coping mechanisms. Survival was the only option and the child that was Emily, along with her feelings, became locked away inside herself, as if in a castle surrounded by a moat; the drawbridge was pulled up and fastened securely. Emily was trying to protect herself. It wasn't going to be effective, but she couldn't know that. She threw away the key.

## FOOD FUSS

Every moment of every day was timetabled, both during the week and at weekends. The girls were woken by a bell; meals, snacks, drinks, baths, prep (homework), letter writing, and shoe cleaning were at fixed times and there were set days for changing clothes and collecting laundry. A member of staff always sat at the end of the table and the girls' places were pre-allocated at the beginning of term. At the opposite end was the 'clearer's' place and the threat was that any food left on the plates had to be eaten by the clearer. Since the girls rotated one space anticlockwise round the table before every meal, cooperation was guaranteed. Emily learnt how to swallow the fat and gristle of the poor-quality meat, as well as mashed swede and rice pudding which she also disliked. But try as she might, she could not eat cheese, which came in many different forms. Every mealtime was a lottery as she struggled to satisfy her hunger when always anxious about what was on the menu. She could smuggle cheese pie out of the dining room in the pocket of the faded blue, long-sleeved overall they wore for meals, but egg in cheese sauce was a real nightmare. One term she sat next to Anne who hated eggs – this suited them both – Anne ate Emily's cheese and Emily ate her eggs.

But inevitably the day came when Emily was caught. It was teatime and Miss Meany dismissed all the other girls except Emily. She sat on the wooden bench on one side of the long, narrow, pine dining table while Miss Meany stood opposite her, glowering. She was not an attractive woman at the best of times, but it was the steely look of her close-set eyes which seemed larger behind the thick lenses of her dark-framed glasses that seemed so oppressive. Emily pushed the cold, congealed cheese sauce around her plate, lifted the fork to her lips, but she couldn't put it in her mouth. Forbidden tears rolled down her cheeks as she sat, unable to look up, continually toying with the thick, off-white mess on the plate. Miss Meany threatened and cajoled, and the clock ticked away during the silence that followed. But try as she might, Miss Meany could not force Emily to eat. Having reached an impasse, Miss Meany let her go but with a firm warning that unless she had a letter from the school doctor, Emily would not get away with it next time.

Sunday, the next letter-writing day, Emily wrote an emotional plea to her mother. It was rewarded when she was seen by the school doctor and after a brief interrogation on why she couldn't eat cheese, he granted her a medical exemption.

It was widely believed that being made to eat everything taught children not to be fussy, but Emily's adult tastes do not bear this out. To this day, she has an aversion to any strong-smelling cheese.

## ALICE

Emily was small for her age and young for her class. For the rest of the year, she was placed in a dormitory with girls from classes below hers. Apparently having lights out fifteen minutes earlier would help her grow, along with the Minadex vitamins she was made to take. Eight-year-old Alice slept in the bed next to Emily and was also homesick. Her home was only a couple of miles away and she couldn't understand why her mother collected her little sister from school every day while she was made to stay. Often Alice complained of tummy ache and frequently she vomited. But Miss Sourpuss berated her. "Alice, you haven't chewed your food properly." Little did they know how it would end for Alice.

## BULLY

Siobhan was a terrible bully who systematically picked on each girl in the dorm, one at a time. Somehow, she managed to coerce the others to join her, as she dreamed up cruel and sometimes violent punishments for her victim. Somehow both Emily and Alice managed to resist, refusing to participate. But Siobhan was a tyrant, forcing her victim to eat soap, or getting the others to set alarms and take shifts to prevent the poor girl from sleeping. She fashioned a whip from stinging nettles and holly and still the terrified victim didn't report what went on, even when the mysterious rash was evident to the matrons and the doctor was called in. She made apple-pie beds, so the sheets got ripped or put spiders in the beds. When she poured water into Emily's bed and demanded that she go and tell the matrons she had wet the bed, Emily finally lost her temper. Although she slept on wet sheets that night, Siobhan left her alone.

The whole dorm was miserable night after night, day after day, always worried about who Siobhan would pick on next and the horrors she had dreamt up. Even though Emily continued to stand her ground, refusing to join in, she couldn't stop it from happening. The only respite came during the few weekends when girls were allowed home for exeats.

Overseas children were forced to stay at school, unless invited out by a friend or relative. On one of these exeats, Sadie invited Emily to come home with her and just before they were due to return to school, Sadie hid herself in the loft and refused to come down. Sadie's father drove Emily back to school on her own and during the journey asked what was going on. Emily told him about the bullying, and he was furious. He asked Emily why *she* hadn't told the matrons. Emily was silent. Why didn't *he* get it? Why couldn't *he* understand that the matrons never listened? Thankfully, he went straight to the headmistress and Siobhan was removed from their dorm. The relief was tangible, not that it changed Emily's feelings about being at school.

## SUPPRESSION

The only way girls could communicate with their families was by post and Emily longed for her mother's letters. They were invariably cheerful, and signed off with the reassurance that it wasn't long until the holidays. Emily no longer wrote about her misery, instead she wracked her brains for things her parents might like to hear. At least they acquiesced when she asked to come home a few days early before the end of term, and return a few days late, after the holidays.

But even if there had been no bullying, or Emily hadn't been forced to eat everything on her plate, or the matrons had been kind, Emily was nine when she went away to school. She was desperately homesick and missed her siblings and her parents. She missed being home. She missed her room, her toys, her pets. There was nobody to talk about how her day had been. There was no adult to help her make sense of what was happening; there was no affection, no love, no kisses, and no goodnight to be had. She longed for the holidays, and nobody understood how unhappy she was or the depths of her despair. It never occurred to her to refuse to go back or to run away from school. She had no control over the situation and no choice other than to carry on. She didn't know of any other way to draw attention to her plight.

The fact that Emily wasn't listened to when she tried asking for help, made it difficult for her to trust anyone. Her parents' good intentions backfired spectacularly. They thought a boarding school education would give her many advantages, but instead it sowed the seeds which ultimately led to a serious mental breakdown, during which she became suicidal and almost lost her life.

Emily's first year at boarding school came to an end and school life began to improve but there was plenty more to endure. It wasn't just the flights to and from Thailand that were long haul.

* * *

*Children are not responsible for the calamities they suffer and anyone brave enough to share what happened needs their story to be validated. Are you a survivor of trauma, abuse, or neglect in childhood?*

*Often those who have survived are asked why they didn't ask for help. Some tried and were not heard; others were so afraid of their abuser(s) that they dare not. Later they may find it difficult to trust others, particularly authority figures. What is your experience?*

# CHAPTER 4

# The school year

Now at boarding school, Emily's life evolved into an endless cycle; during term time she crossed days off on a homemade calendar counting down to the holidays, but once back at home the initial euphoria was short-lived. Within forty-eight hours, the dread of the impending return to school started and hung over her like an ever-approaching storm.

Just as Emily started boarding school, the Foreign Office unexpectedly closed the consulate in Chiang Mai. George was redeployed to the British Embassy in Bangkok and oversaw the Queen's visit to Thailand, for which he was later awarded the MVO.

## PERFECT PARENTS

Emily's parents were still perfect in her eyes, before adolescent disillusionment set in. Jane, her talented mother, regularly exhibited and sold her batik artwork. She was also a published writer, although as a diplomat's wife, she concealed her identity with different pen names. She wrote for the magazine *Punch*, a column for the *Daily Telegraph* and was the author of a very successful play, performed the world over. Later, one of her books was published by Victor Gollancz. Yet Jane underrated her own achievements and frequently lamented her lack of a university education.

Emily admired her so much and wanted to be like her, but more than anything she wanted to please her. Unlike her glamorous mother, Emily wasn't especially pretty. Jane used to apologise that Emily had inherited her fine hair and often commented on how unphotogenic she was. But George and Jane were clear that the ultimate goal for all of their children was that of academic achievement and a place at university. Emily wasn't doing well at school with the exception of story writing. She also excelled at diving, swimming, and gymnastics, all of which became displacement activities as she still secretly harboured the dream of becoming a ballet dancer.

## NO ACQUITTAL

It was two years since the lying incident, but Emily still felt guilty. She wanted to come clean to her parents and during the holidays lay awake rehearsing what she was going to say, all to the hum of the air-conditioner. Finally, she managed to pluck up courage, crept downstairs to the living room and hastily blurted out her confession. Jane put down her book, smiled and calmly said, "It's all right, Emily, you were young. Be a good girl and go back to bed."

It was such an anticlimax! Emily had just offloaded her deepest, darkest secret and she didn't feel any better. But it was even more difficult to vocalise her unhappiness when her parents repeatedly reminded her how lucky she was to be at boarding school. As the end of the holidays approached, Emily couldn't hold back the tears while she reluctantly packed her suitcase for the eighteen-hour flight back to London. She cried so much during the journey that it upset the other passengers; the air hostess moved her to the curtained-off area for the crew at the back of the plane.

Someone must have let her parents know because from the next holiday, the local doctor prescribed tranquillisers to sedate her for subsequent flights back to England. At least it helped Emily sleep through those miserable plane journeys.

Decades later, Jane revealed that they assumed Emily was fine once she arrived back at school. But like most boarding school survivors, Emily retreated back into her survival mode during term time; she became detached, her emotions suppressed, tears hidden, aware only of her deep, inner misery.

## SENIORS

After two years, Emily's class moved up to senior school. No longer watched over by the junior school's vindictive matrons, the girls were freed from many of the draconian rules. Daily life improved but Emily's homesickness did not. Academically she was far from thriving, streamed to the bottom group for Latin and Maths, middle group for everything else. The only subject where she consistently excelled was English. Her end of term report stated, '*Emily has a very vivid imagination*' – it didn't seem to be a good thing.

## PLANE CRASH

In the Easter holidays of 1972, when Emily was twelve, Jane flew back to see Andrew and Emily for the unfunded third holiday of the year. They were staying with their maternal grandparents in Devon before term started when the BBC broadcast news of a plane crash in Addis Ababa. Emily was shocked and astonished to see the headshot of her school friend Diana on the television. Back at school, their class was assembled together to hear news directly from Diana's uncle. Diana had been flown back to RAF Brize Norton, along with the other surviving British casualties and was now in hospital receiving treatment for serious burns. He described her bravery as she tried to help her friend Caroline who had been sitting next to her on the plane. Sadly, Caroline, who was also twelve years old, subsequently died from her injuries. Before the class was dismissed, they were told not to talk about it anymore and on no account to question Diana about the crash once she was well enough to return to school.

It is very unlikely that Emily was the only one who felt overwhelmed by the tragedy, but she thought she had no right to feel the way she did – after all, it was not her friend who died, and she was not the one who had survived a plane crash! But Emily couldn't stop thinking about it, wondering why it happened and how Diana would ever be able to get on a plane again. There were so many unanswered questions. But they were used to doing as they were told and didn't talk about their feelings. Life just carried on, as it always did.

Diana did return to school towards the end of term, and Emily was in awe of her fortitude and cheerfulness. Through all the years that followed, Emily never lost her admiration or forgot about her. It didn't seem surprising that Diana was made head girl several years later.

In 2021, on the way to work, I tuned in to *Life Changing* on BBC Radio 4. The guest on the programme was Harriet Ware-Austin, and I was stunned to hear her giving her own account of how she had witnessed that very same plane crash from the viewing platform at the airport in Addis Ababa. Harriet's two older sisters were also on the way back to school in England on that fateful day and it was her sister – twelve-year-old Caroline, who sat next to Diana on the plane. At take-off, the plane hit a piece of debris on the runway and skidded off course when a tyre burst. It then crashed down an embankment at the end of the runway, before bursting into flames. Tragically, forty-three of the passengers lost their lives, including both of Harriet's sisters, Jane and Caroline. It was incredibly moving to listen to Harriet's heart-breaking account of the tragedy. There was a tremendous response to the broadcast, from the friends and family who had never had the chance to find out what happened or to talk about it. Harriet received many messages from people who expressed their gratitude because it enabled them to speak openly about their loss for the first time. The silence that had prevailed was so typical of the seventies and at last the embargo surrounding this tragic event was lifted.

Harriet's account touched me deeply and I found myself sobbing my heart out. The confusion and mystery around the plane crash was over and the emotions buried for so long finally surfaced. A memorial plaque to the passengers and crew who lost their lives was unveiled at the British Embassy in Ethiopia in 2022. Many of those who died were children on their way back to boarding school.

## BROKEN ARM

During that summer of 1972, Emily fell and broke her arm. It was Friday and the matron bandaged her arm with cotton wool soaked in witch-hazel and put it in a sling. They didn't take her to hospital until Monday. X-rays confirmed fractures at the wrist and elbow. There was no anaesthetic when they manipulated her fracture. The nurses held Emily down while she kicked and screamed. Afterwards she was taken back to school and put to bed in sick bay. She lay by herself in the small room watching the white curtains with little pink flowers gently move in the breeze. She couldn't eat when the matron brought in the supper. How could she sleep when all she knew was that tomorrow she had to go back to the hospital? Her heart raced at the thought.

All was well at the review appointment; she was just there to have the plaster cast completed. It was such a relief to get back to class and submit to the pleasing ritual of having the plaster signed by friends. But Josephine was having none of it.

"Why are you wearing a sling? You're a hypochondriac. When I broke my arm in the holidays, they took me to the operating theatre!"

Emily's cast extended above her elbow fixing it at a right angle; nonetheless she discarded the sling straight away, rather than endure the contemptuous allegation levelled at girls who made too much fuss. How could she possibly articulate the torture she'd been through at the hospital?

## FAILED ESCAPE PLAN

Hannah had a desk in front of Emily and spent hours and hours in the classroom, staying late after prep (homework) had finished. It wasn't just that she was working hard, Emily could see how odd Hannah's writing had become; the words on one side of the page were huge and then got progressively smaller until they were tiny at the other. Then one day Hannah was summoned to see the headmistress and sent home.

Perfect! Emily now knew what she had to do. She stayed late in the classroom every evening, burying herself in her studies, intent on 'overdoing it'. It was the very first time that Emily made any sustained effort over her schoolwork, but she decided not to copy Hannah's strange writing, fearing it might make her plans too obvious.

Then at last, she was called to Miss Brown's office. The headmistress had a spacious study overlooking the lawn, with carpets on the floor, furnished as a comfortable sitting room, possibly designed to put prospective parents at ease. Miss Brown commended Emily for the way her marks had suddenly improved. As a result, she was now going to be moved up to the top groups for all subjects. She dismissed Emily and it was only as she was going through the door that Miss Brown called after her, "but don't work *too* hard."

Emily was devastated. She was not being sent home, and worse still, she now had to be in classes with all the brainy girls. How was she ever going to keep up with them? She went to find Mrs Drinkwater, her Latin teacher. Surely, she knew it would be much better for her to stay in the bottom group. But Mrs Drinkwater was no help at all, she said Emily needed to be stretched.

## MISERY REVEALED

The consulate in Chiang Mai was reopened and Emily's father took up his commission as the British Consul. Andrew and Emily joined their family that summer, in the most beautiful colonial house situated on the banks of the Mae Ping River. The weather was much more temperate than Bangkok and the surrounding hills and jungle were enigmatic. At the end of the holidays Emily's father accompanied her as far as Bangkok, where she would catch the connecting flight back to London. George witnessed for himself the way she cried throughout the whole journey and by the time they parted company as Emily went through to the international departure lounge, he was also in tears. Maybe this was what provoked the decision to move Emily to a different school.

## UNTIMELY DEATH

Meanwhile Emily arrived back for her fourth consecutive year at boarding school, to learn that her young friend Alice, had gone into a coma and died on the first day of the holidays. Emily was stunned. Poor, unhappy Alice was dead. She found a place in the middle of a wooded area in the school grounds, where rhododendron bushes formed a shield around her. Unobserved, she sat on a tree stump to cry, utterly bewildered, unable to make sense of it all.

For many years I wondered whether Alice would still be alive if she'd been given more attention. It was not reassuring as a medical student to discover that her symptoms of abdominal pain and vomiting were often the first signs of diabetes in children. Hoping to put an end to such speculation, I viewed Alice's death certificate which is in the public domain; it confirmed my worst fears – she died in a hyperglycaemic coma from undiagnosed diabetes. The words *'no inquest required'* had been written at the top of the death certificate. So, there was no investigation to establish for how long Alice had been ill, or whether anything could have been done to prevent her death. She died during an era when little attention was paid to child welfare or child protection, and too many adults were able to hurt or neglect children without any comeback.

## STRIVING

Ironically, during the rest of that school year, Emily finally started to settle. She had discovered the antidote to misery was to bury herself in hard work. When she consistently achieved high marks, her teachers were pleased with her, and she received affirmation as her reward. Striving and diligence became cemented as a coping mechanism for stress and misery. The underlying homesickness was still there, but school became more tolerable.

When her parents suggested a change of school might make her happier, initially Emily agreed but for completely different reasons. She simply wanted to do ballet and that wasn't offered at her current school.

There were practical reasons why Emily's parents chose the next school near to their English home. Her father's tour of duty in Chiang Mai was almost over and in a couple of years, a home posting was expected. Margaret would be due to start secondary school, and it would be far more convenient to have both daughters nearby to take them out for weekends and holidays. Andrew was starting university, and if Emily moved schools, it would avoid any long trips to Bristol.

By the time Emily realised a change of school was a bad idea, her parents said it was too late. Emily was completely unprepared for yet another devastating new experience.

* * *

*In the 1970s showing sadness, misery or grief was often frowned upon. Yet adults seemed to show little restraint when they directed their contempt, disgust, or anger towards children. The results of suppressed emotion are not always obvious, but it may restrain development, and/or creativity in children, as well as become the driving force behind life's future choices. Without role models it may be difficult for people to be open with those closest to them, and may jeopardise significant family relationships in the future. How was it for you? Are you aware of feelings which have been hidden away for years on end?*

# CHAPTER 5

# Changes

The fabric of the new school, like the uniform, was outdated. Originally one large Victorian house, the main school had been extended and converted. The classrooms were small, and the desks looked like they had been rescued from the Dickens era. It was September 1973 and Emily's parents fell off the pedestal. She was thirteen, a turbulent adolescent who was now angry and deeply hurt by what she perceived as their heartlessness.

## BETRAYAL

The first term was the penultimate year before O levels (GCSEs) and her whole year group consisted of about twenty girls; they were taught as one class rather than streamed according to academic ability. Emily had been prepared to sit her Maths O level a year early, but the new school couldn't accommodate that.

Emily wore a gym skirt to her first PE lesson, the one item of compatible school uniform from her previous school. The teacher noticed the badges awarded for gymnastics. "What are those?" she snapped, "get them off by next lesson."

It did not augur well and nothing, it seemed, could mitigate this disastrous change. Friendships in her class were already well established. There was no orchestra, no choir, not even a library and Emily felt like a complete outsider.

Only a few pupils lived overseas and though Emily's family were middle class and certainly not poor, the difference in their social standing was obvious. At her previous school, there were many girls with government-funded places either from Foreign Office or army families; here she was amongst the daughters of the wealthy upper classes. Many in her year were being prepared to 'come out' as debutantes, something Emily knew absolutely nothing about. Few of them had any interest in a career or a place at university.

She couldn't understand why on earth her parents had chosen this school. But she knew she had agreed to move school when they first raised the idea, all motivated by her ridiculous longing to do ballet which had now evaporated in a puff of smoke.

## REGULATIONS

The school regime was characterised by petty and draconian rules. Baths were timetabled three times a week and hair washing was only allowed once a week which was a nightmare for adolescent girls with greasy hair. The only time Emily found sufficient privacy to cry was when she was alone in the bathtub, where she wept buckets, unseen and unheard, finally emerging with her wet hair in a shower cap as she tried to hide her obvious infraction of the rules.

Emily, like her family, had no time for religion, but attendance at church and chapel was mandatory. The girls even had to wear a separate Sunday uniform. The dated language and the constant moralising during tedious sermons seemed both irrelevant and boring.

## BORN-AGAIN BAPTIST

Emily's uncle, John, was a Baptist minister who lived in South London, and he invited her to stay for the precious weekends and half term when she was allowed out of school. Her cousin Julia was just a year older, and they soon became good friends. It was going well until Sunday, when Emily was mortified to find she was obliged to attend church with them.

Despite her misgivings, Emily was surprised at how engaging Uncle John was and found herself listening as he preached a typical evangelical gospel message. Emily had just turned fourteen and knew absolutely nothing about the bible but she needed no convincing to believe she was a sinner. When Uncle John led the congregation in prayer asking God to take away guilt and shame, she silently echoed his words to commit her life to Jesus.

After the service, she felt as if a burden had lifted and the old feeling of guilt over the 'lying incident' had dissipated. Uncle John was thrilled that Emily wanted to be baptised. He went through a pamphlet with her, just to be certain that she fully understood that she was now a born-again Christian.

Emily was even happier when Uncle John asked the headmistress to grant permission for her to have extra weekends out of school, ostensibly to prepare for baptism. This marked the very beginning of Emily's long affiliation with evangelical Christianity.

Uncle John was so delighted by Emily's conversion, and it made her feel special. She enjoyed spending time with his family, even though it was very different from her own. His house was very busy with the coming and going of people from the church congregation. Emily's aunt was very hospitable, and they didn't fuss over their appearance or what was on the menu. It felt relaxing to be there with her cousins.

Emily listened carefully when Uncle John explained the

gospel to her. He said that only the 'saved' would go to heaven after they died, the rest of humankind was destined for hell unless they accepted Jesus as their Lord and saviour. When Emily heard this, she was filled with anxiety, as she contemplated the fate of her own family. Uncle John said she needed to pray for them. Yet Emily couldn't understand why God had chosen her out of the blue but couldn't do the same for everyone else. Uncle John gave her a bible and instructed her to read a passage every day. He reiterated the importance of 'witnessing', which meant she must share her new-found faith with her classmates and then when she went home, with her own family.

Back at school, some of Emily's classmates were preparing for confirmation in the Anglican church. They weren't impressed by Emily's version of Christianity. They had been brought up as Christians and they didn't seem to take their faith nearly so seriously as the Baptists.

The following weekend, Emily related her confusion to her uncle. He explained that those who had been 'born again' were the true believers, but there were others, just 'nominal' Christians, like the girls at school.

Emily was a vulnerable, unhappy teenager, who desperately craved love. She deferred to his opinion – he was the one adult who paid attention to her and took her seriously. Although she didn't dare admit to him that she wasn't going to do any more witnessing either at school or to her family.

Uncle John encouraged Emily to see God's overarching purpose in her life which gave a different perspective to the unhappy change of school; after all, it had led to her salvation! But Emily was over the moon when he asked if she would like to come and live with them and attend a local school like her cousins. Emily's parents said no. Apparently the Foreign Office would not pay for flights to visit them in the holidays unless she was at boarding school; the matter was closed.

## FRAGILE FAMILY RELATIONSHIPS

Although on some level, Emily's new faith helped her cope, it also put her own family relationships in jeopardy. When she flew back to Chiang Mai for the Christmas holidays, she discovered that her parents were not overly happy with her conversion to Christianity. Her mother described how some of the local missionaries had parked outside the consulate during one of their parties and deliberately blared Christian music as a sign of their censure. Emily agreed this was both rude and disrespectful as her mother pointed out the arrogance of Christians who thought of themselves as better than everyone else. She realised she had to tread carefully, but it did nothing to relieve her anxiety; Emily fretted over how her family might die and not go to heaven. She realised she wasn't really part of Uncle John's family, but now her faith made her feel isolated even in her own home.

## THE MISSIONARY

Around this time Emily decided she wanted to become a doctor. Not only did her parents find this acceptable, it also fitted the Christian ethos perfectly. Uncle John suggested that she meet a friend of his. Jasper was a missionary surgeon who worked at the university hospital in Chiang Mai. During the Easter holidays of 1975, Jasper came to the consulate to fetch Emily. He was tall and lean, with piercing blue eyes. He instructed her to put her arms around his waist for support as they sped off on his motorbike without wearing helmets. First, Jasper took Emily on one of his missionary visits, accompanied by his wife and young children. It was interesting to walk through the paddy fields to reach the remote Thai village, but it was hot and boring to be sat in the sultry humidity of a villager's wooden house without the luxury of a fan. Emily's Thai wasn't good enough to understand the discussion, but she sensed that the villager's response to Jasper's discourse was far from enthusiastic.

The second time Emily met Jasper, he had invited her to observe his work at the hospital. It was an exciting morning as she watched him operate, and then afterwards, Jasper took Emily to see a male patient. Apparently, the man's wife couldn't get pregnant, and Jasper needed a 'sample' to diagnose the cause of their infertility. Emily was fourteen, very naïve and had no idea what this entailed. When Jasper asked if she would like to watch, she assumed it would be something like a blood test. Just before she was due to go into the tiny room with the patient, Jasper said he needed a quick word with him first. It was only when Emily caught sight of his face, that she realised something was terribly wrong. She felt so stupid as it dawned on her what she had agreed to. She fled from the hospital determined never to see Jasper again. Embarrassed and ashamed, she didn't dare breathe a word about it to anyone.

## POSSIBLE RHEUMATIC FEVER

In the autumn term of her O level year, having just turned fifteen, Emily was taken ill. She was still very unhappy at school, and as usual coped by burying herself in her studies. One day, her arms and legs started to tremble. It grew steadily worse until she was shaking uncontrollably. Feverish, she was admitted to a private hospital which didn't normally take children. The doctors kept doing ECGs and repeatedly listening to her racing heart. They kept telling her to try and keep still, but she couldn't control her trembling limbs. The doctors suspected 'St Vitus' Dance', an unusual manifestation of rheumatic fever. The nurses raised the bed rails and lined them with pillows to prevent Emily's flailing limbs from hitting the sides. After ten days or so, her condition improved but a neurologist had been asked to see her. He asked about school, and Emily readily admitted her misery.

Emily was discharged into Uncle John's care and the church prayed for her healing. The shaking certainly improved but every time she was anxious, she tried to hide a slight tremor which surfaced again. Once Emily was well enough to return to school, she found she didn't have enough energy to catch up on the schoolwork she had missed.

In the Christmas holidays, Emily's worried parents wanted a second opinion from a local doctor in Chiang Mai. They wondered whether her illness had been Dengue fever which was endemic in the area, but Emily had seen the letter from the neurologist on her mother's desk: *'Emily will stop shaking when she wants to.'* How could she trust anyone when they obviously thought she had made up her symptoms? Emily refused point blank to see any more doctors who might blame her for being ill.

## MEDIOCRITY

Up until the time of her illness, Emily had been doing very well academically. She had come top of her class and scored one hundred per cent in the Maths exam. But now she had lost all momentum and fallen way behind. Even with O levels pending, Emily's parents decided she wasn't well enough to return to school and postponed her return flight.

Perhaps it was the relief of being allowed to stay at home that renewed Emily's verve and enthusiasm. She scoured the English library for books on subjects she was studying and took French lessons at the Alliance Française.

She met a Lisu-hill-tribe student who had a scholarship to study French, and they became friends. The day he asked Emily to marry him, he brought her a present of dried opium poppies from his village – she was amused and flattered, but her father didn't see the funny side of it and sent him packing.

Emily was given a choice: either she had to go back to school and take her exams or give up all ideas of becoming a doctor.

She tried to persuade her parents to let her finish her O levels by correspondence course, but they were adamant. Jane reminded Emily of her own regret at leaving school aged sixteen and how she was unable to go to university as a result. It felt like Hobson's choice and reluctantly Emily capitulated. It was a struggle to get through to the end of the year and Emily's O level results were mediocre at best.

## INSTITUTIONAL INADEQUACY

In the sixth form, Emily discovered she didn't even have the necessary subjects to apply to medical school and she had to teach Emily and herself to get her Physics and Chemistry O levels. So much for this expensive education. Her school didn't teach A level Chemistry either, so Emily had to cycle to a neighbouring school for these vital classes.

The school had little to offer in music either, but Emily found solace in playing the clarinet. The peripatetic teacher, who was also a bandsman in the Blues and Royals, came to teach Emily and the only other pupil who played a wind instrument. He was very enthusiastic, friendly, and encouraging – and another man whose interest in young women was far from benign. He promised to reward Emily for her hard work by taking her out to a concert, but it had to wait until she was a student in London. He assured Emily that he often met up with his ex-pupils and it seemed a nice idea.

Finally, A levels were finished, and news came that she had made the grades for medical school. It was liberating. Despite eight miserable years of boarding school and everything life had thrown at her, she had survived.

* * *

*Undoubtedly many children and young people cope well despite dire circumstances. Yet low-level, unremitting adversity can be profoundly damaging and have repercussions later in life. Even though your childhood may have been completely different, is there anything in your early life which resonates with Emily's experiences?*

# CHAPTER 6

# Life as a medical student

Emily was almost eighteen when she started at St George's Medical School, in London. All British university students were eligible for a means-tested government grant, which paid their fees and funded their living expenses. It was a great leveller, putting students on a par, as far as their income was concerned. Emily revelled in the freedom, at last able to choose what she did and when.

## RE-ENCOUNTERING CHRISTIANITY

During her first week at St George's, a fourth-year student, Edward, introduced himself. He went to a local Baptist church on Sundays and the minister was Emily's very own Uncle John; he had asked Edward to look out for her. This took Emily by surprise. She hadn't had any contact with her uncle over the last couple of years, nor was she familiar with the geography of London. She didn't know that St George's was only five miles away from his church.

Edward was also president of the CU (Christian Union) and invited Emily to join them. Although Emily had largely forgotten about her Christian faith during the intervening years, she thought it was the most extraordinary coincidence that this had happened and a sign of Divine providence.

The CU members were enthusiastic and keen to evangelise their peers. It felt as though Emily's newly acquired freedom had shrunk a little, but she did her best to conform to the Christian philosophy and lifestyle, which the other CU students embraced so readily. Before long, Emily felt disappointed that the 'Christian' way of life wasn't all it was cracked out to be. Assuming it was because she was so new to Christianity, she bought a bible and threw herself heart and soul into the activities organised by the CU, determined to try harder to be committed to God.

## PREDATOR

Nonetheless, the first year at medical school was really enjoyable; Emily found plenty of interests, helped set up the medical school orchestra and joined one of the London choirs. Her parents left for a posting in Brunei, and she hardly noticed their departure. The clarinet teacher made good on his promise, and Emily dressed up ready for an entertaining evening out. He was a good-looking man in his late thirties, clean-shaven, dark hair, smart in his jacket and tie. He treated Emily to a sumptuous dinner before the concert. Afterwards he drove her back to the student halls and just before Emily opened the car door, she felt a hand on her thigh. She didn't ask him in for coffee and predictably never heard from him again.

## BRUNEI SUMMER

After first-year exams, Emily joined her parents in Brunei, for the long summer vacation. Their house had a beautiful view over the estuary, the climate was hot and the town was interesting. But Emily didn't know anyone, and she didn't know how to fill her time. When she heard that a British doctor wanted some help with his research, she jumped at the chance. He worked at the hospital in Bandar Seri Begawan, and wanted to investigate the nutritional status of local pregnant women. He asked Emily to learn enough Malay to pose simple questions about diet and taught her how to take blood samples. Then the real work began as she accompanied the midwives to antenatal clinics, often leaving at first light to travel by boat to reach longhouses in remote jungle areas. On return to base, Emily then became the lab technician, and was taught how to process the blood samples they had taken. It was interesting, but she was unpaid, and it was hard work. When her vacation drew to a close, this doctor still wanted more from her. He asked Emily to get the results analysed back at medical school, having devised some strange mathematical algorithms which he was sure would prove his theories about nutrition. By this time Emily was reluctant to agree but couldn't refuse him either. Admittedly she didn't understand what he was trying to do, but she was just a student. He was the qualified doctor and she figured he knew best.

Back at St George's, Emily sought the help of one of her lecturers. He was extremely kind to Emily but completely frank as he blew holes in the Brunei doctor's research methodology, as well as his theories. It was disappointing to find that the months she had spent as an unpaid lackey had been a complete waste of time. The only solace was that it had been a great experience to be able to visit some of the indigenous people who still lived in relatively inaccessible communities.

## DISENCHANTED

During the second year at medical school, Emily felt lonely; it worried her that she hadn't had a boyfriend yet. The CU maintained that intimate relationships must only be with fellow Christians and there was a strictly 'no sex before marriage' ethos. Secretly Emily thought it was most unfair, especially since there were far more single women than men within church circles. She decided to seek the wisdom of one of the church elders. But Don infuriated her further, when he told her that she shouldn't be looking for a boyfriend – what she really needed was a husband. Emily's patience was wearing thin; she thought these Christians were out of touch with reality and resented their overly pious attitudes.

Just before the summer vacation Emily arranged to flat-share with two male students in her year, neither of whom were Christians. They found a three-bedroom flat on the top floor of a typical multi-occupancy house. One of her flatmates, Paul, was extremely clever but not at all ostentatious. He also seemed a bit of a rebel, unbothered by rules and regulations. He knew a lot about cars and engines, just the person to have around with Emily's temperamental motorbike. When some of the CU made it known that they were not happy with her future living arrangements, Emily left the CU.

She did well in her second-year exams and was offered a Medical Research Council grant to do an additional year for an intercalated BSc. Although it meant being alone all summer, she couldn't face another long vacation in Brunei and arranged to visit her parents at Christmas instead.

## SUMMER VACATION

During the summer vacation Emily found a job as a mortuary assistant at one of the local hospitals. Liam, the senior mortuary attendant, was a wiry man in his thirties who spent most of the day at 'Ivy Cottage' doing the crossword with Radio 1 blasting loudly in the background. He tolerated Emily, as a rather tiresome encumbrance to his solitary job, only motivated because it seemed that death wasn't seasonal enough to give him a summer holiday. He had to teach Emily to take responsibility for preparing bodies for post-mortems, which she relished as worthy education for a medical student. But most of the time, there wasn't much to do, and she sat reading a novel, disturbed only occasionally to answer the phone or to open the door to the porters with their macabre deliveries. The Irish pathologist, Dr O'Toole, had a great sense of humour and enjoyed giving Emily ad hoc teaching while he carried out the post-mortems. His enthusiasm was infectious, and Emily thought that if she stayed much longer, he would persuade her into a career in pathology.

On Sundays during the summer, Emily went along to the service at the Baptist church and sat with the St George's clinical students who no longer had the luxury of the long vacation. They invited her to the Proms at the Royal Albert Hall and later one afternoon, she found herself walking beside one of their flatmates. Peter was a trainee programmer working for the NHS. He had long, dark, wavy hair down to his shoulders and a full beard, a sort of cultivated hippy look, with holes in his jeans and frayed bottoms. Emily couldn't stop thinking about him and decided to risk dropping by his flat one evening after work. She was happy when he invited her for lunch the following Sunday and despite the butterflies in her stomach, she could hardly wait.

It was disastrous to find how badly she had misread the situation. There were some other female guests who seemed to be well acquainted with Peter. As they had to leave straight after lunch, Peter suggested they all walk to the Tube station together since it was a beautiful, warm, August day. Still feeling deflated, Emily was tempted to make her excuses, but she was curious, and not yet ready to give up her hopes.

## BOYFRIEND

After they had said their goodbyes, Peter and Emily ambled slowly across Clapham Common and suddenly she felt him take her hand in his. They spent the rest of the day together, talking for hours. The following week, they met every day after work and spent every opportunity they could in each other's company. Emily was madly in love and couldn't believe how lucky she was. Her boyfriend was different to most men she knew; Peter was kind, sensitive and thoughtful. Although quietly spoken, he knew his mind.

Three weeks after they started going out, Peter invited her to come with him to meet his parents. It was a little nerve-wracking knowing that his mother was a doctor, but she needn't have worried, Kay was the perfect hostess. Peter's father said very little, but his wife made up for it with lots of chatter and constant laughter. As they waited on the platform for the train back to London, Peter turned to Emily. "Do you think we will ever get married?"

She shrugged, not sure quite how to reply. "What do you think?"

"I'm asking you," he said.

"Yes," she answered breathlessly.

Later that night as Emily lay in bed alone in her flat, she felt as though Christmas had come. It was hard to grasp that Peter loved her enough to want to spend the rest of his life with her after such a short time. Incredible! Then doubt crept in. Surely this was foolhardy. Her Christian friends would never do anything so rash; they would have prayed about it, 'waited on the Lord'. They frequently seemed to need the Almighty's approval for even the smallest decisions, let alone momentous, life-changing ones. Then she remembered Don's words – hadn't he told her to look for a husband? Emily dismissed her momentary concerns. She was head over heels in love with Peter and it was only natural to be a little nervous. This was happening to her, the unlovable one who had never had a boyfriend!

## FIANCÉ

When the summer was over, most of Emily's medical student peers progressed to the three years of clinical studies on the wards, while she started her intercalated BSc. Peter and Emily had decided to delay the announcement of their engagement until they had told Emily's parents. They were due back on leave the following summer which seemed perfect timing for a wedding, so Emily wrote asking if she could bring Peter to spend Christmas with them in Brunei.

Emily's parents had never been very tolerant over the way 'young people dressed nowadays' and her father had a particular dislike of long hair and beards. Peter made an effort to smarten up, cut his hair a bit shorter, and trimmed his beard but Emily didn't kid herself that it would be enough.

The weather in Brunei was hot, and they had some delightful trips to the beach and an adventurous trip with an army helicopter to visit a remote longhouse. Christmas came and went, but Peter and Emily hadn't plucked up courage to broach the subject of their engagement. On New Year's Eve, sitting beneath the whirring fan, they finally shared their plans. Emily had prepared herself for the inevitability of George and Jane's objections but not for their silence.

On New Year's Day, the whole family took a trip to one of the islands off the coast, waterskiing and snorkelling. Emily tried to break the impasse by asking her two younger sisters to be her bridesmaids but still her parents made no comment about their plans to get married.

The morning before Peter and Emily's flight back to England, they were in town doing some shopping and Emily commented on some cute baby clothes she saw on one of the displays. Jane stiffly reminded her that babies should be the last thing on her mind. Finally, Jane broke the ice before they left, suggesting to Emily that they might try living together, instead of marrying. Emily didn't have the courage to tell her that effectively, they were doing so already.

## ANNOUNCEMENT

Back in England, Peter's parents' reaction to their news could hardly have been more different. Champagne was brought out and without hesitation Kay started planning the wedding cake and brought out her pattern books, determined that she would assist in making the dresses. Emily was overwhelmed with gratitude that they were so positive about it all.

Peter received a letter from Emily's parents saying they would not be prepared to support *his* wife through the rest of her medical school training. He replied straight away, saying it was perfectly all right, because he planned to give Emily all the support she needed. Almost by return of post, Emily's parents sent a cheque towards the cost of the wedding. It seemed that Peter's declaration had soothed their unspoken fears.

At the time, Emily felt hurt, unable to see her parents' point of view or understand their legitimate concerns over her future career. She was only twenty and they didn't know that their future son-in-law was all they could have wished for. Peter was sensible, upright, and hard-working and had no intention of taking Emily away from her career. It wasn't until she was a parent of adult children herself, that Emily understood some of their concerns. But she fared little better, also failing to have proper conversations with her own children over important issues. Retrospect makes it easy to identify mistakes but it's challenging to break the habits passed down through the generations. Emily's family were not the only ones unaccustomed to talking things through. It was a common enough legacy from their culture.

As summer exams approached, Emily tried to revise for her BSc finals, admittedly distracted by the wedding preparations. After the results came out, she met with her tutor for the last time. He told her how she stood out from the other candidates but cautioned that it was neither a compliment nor an insult. The examiners noted how she had given an exceptional degree of thought to her answers both in the written papers and in the *viva voce*, but "they lacked fact". Emily was very happy to be awarded a 2:1 (upper second-class degree).

## WEDDING

The weather was perfect, beautifully sunny and hot on her wedding day. George proudly walked her down the aisle and later at the self-catered reception held in the medical school bar, he stood on an upturned bottle crate to give a moving father-of-the-bride speech. It seemed that Emily's parents had abandoned their misgivings, and subsequently they invited the newlyweds to join them on a holiday in France after their honeymoon.

* * *

*Patterns of behaviour may be established in early life and follow into adulthood. Emily was able to hold her own most of the time, but had developed a tendency to defer to experts, especially male authority figures. Can you distinguish which of your traits are helpful from those which may be a hindrance? Can you see any patterns in the way you respond to people or situations?*

# CHAPTER 7

# Married at medical school

September 1980 brought Emily back to reality as she started her full-time clinical training for her final three years of medical school. Medical students were split into small, self-selected groups called firms as they rotated through the various specialities learning the basics of medical practice. Written finals were scheduled for October 1982 and then the final examinations to assess their clinical skills would take place later in June 1983. The newly qualified doctors were then expected to start work on August 1st to do their 'housejobs', the pre-registration year.

## BABY TALK

Peter and Emily had moved to a ground-floor bedsit, rented from Emily's previous landlord. The condition of the property left a lot to be desired, but at least they had a gas fire and they decided to get a kitten to deal with the infestation of mice.

They joined a 'house group' at the church, where they met other young couples. Emily was happy as they began to assimilate within the church community, but Peter was more reticent when it came to accepting all the Baptist church teachings. Many of their friends had babies and young children and Emily began to feel broody. But Peter agreed with Jane, now was not the time to start a family.

## GUINEA PIG

Peter had completed his training and worked for the NHS as a computer programmer, nonetheless money was tight. Emily saw a flyer on the medical school noticeboard, advertising for volunteers to participate in obesity research. They were looking for 'lean' controls and participants would receive a £70 honorarium which would be a welcome contribution to household expenses.

The researchers were pretty nonchalant and gave no warnings about the dangers of the proposed insulin stress test, where participants would lose consciousness as their blood sugars plummeted. Another test involved the infusion of noradrenalin, and it was all to take place in the lab block, without facilities for resuscitation. Since they were qualified doctors, Emily assumed they knew exactly what they were doing and that it was all perfectly safe. As part of the project, participants would need to double their calorie intake; they were warned that even with the addition of specially prepared milkshakes to their diet, it would not be as easy as it sounds. When Emily felt nauseous the whole time and had lots of nightmares, she was reassured it was to be expected. But as Emily walked across the covered walkway to the lab block for the second of the insulin stress tests, she noticed her breasts felt tender. A fleeting thought crossed her mind – *maybe I'm pregnant*. She was on the contraceptive pill and dismissed it. A couple of days later, after the very unpleasant insulin stress test, she returned for the noradrenalin infusion.

As it was proceeding, one of the researchers suddenly leapt to his feet because Emily's heart had gone into a dangerous rhythm. Thankfully it reverted to normal once the infusion was stopped, but they seemed very shaken by what happened and paid Emily the full honorarium, asking her not to return to complete the remaining tests.

Not long after, Emily started to bleed heavily. When she passed a small but recognisable foetus, it felt as if the world had stopped. Not unreasonably, she leapt to the conclusion that the miscarriage was a direct result of the low blood sugar caused by the insulin stress test. She berated herself as she recalled the fleeting moment when she thought she might be pregnant. Overwhelmed with guilt and grief she blamed herself for killing her unborn baby for the paltry sum of £70. It never occurred to her that the researchers had a duty of care, nor that she had been subjected to unethical and dangerous tests without informed consent. Today such research would never pass ethics committee approval.

## MISCARRIAGE

Peter knew about the miscarriage, but Emily couldn't bring herself to admit that she felt responsible. When Emily saw her GP, he said it was just as well because she couldn't continue medical school while pregnant. Emily burst into tears and fled from his surgery. She ran through Tooting in panic, believing there was no one to turn to. She thought her medical school friends would concur with the GP and she couldn't tell her pro-life church friends since the miscarriage was her own fault. Too ashamed to confess the truth to anyone, Emily needed to get a grip on herself.

Finally, she found the strength and told herself to carry on, just as she had done before so many times while growing up and it was best not to make any fuss. For the next thirty years,

Emily buried the memory. The overwhelming shame had felt too unbearable to contemplate.

It doesn't take much to opine that it was Emily's unresolved grief that drove her increasing desire to have a baby. While still at medical school and without family support, logically, Emily knew it was utterly foolish, yet she deliberately chose to be careless with contraception.

## STREATHAM

Peter and Emily moved to a little terraced house round the corner from the church in South London. It was further from St George's, but it was good to be away from the main road. Their beloved cat Wellie had already lost one of his nine lives, breaking a leg in the process. The house was a classic two-up two-down, which had never been modernised; there was an outside toilet, and a bath located in the kitchen, with a tabletop fitted over it – also the only surface which could be used to prepare food. The small boiler fed water into an unlagged tank which gave enough hot water for the kitchen sink and one bath. The only source of heating was a gas fire in the downstairs living room, but Peter and Emily loved it. Their house-group leaders lived just a five-minute walk away and Emily felt part of the church community.

## PREGNANT

It was spring in her penultimate year of medical school when Emily started feeling nauseous and couldn't stand the smell of coffee. When a friend suggested she might be pregnant, she vehemently denied it. But the next day, she went to the chemist and handed in her urine sample for a pregnancy test. During the delay waiting for the result, she went up the high street and bought herself a tight-fitting dress as though it could stop it all from happening.

The positive test threw Emily into turmoil, and she called Peter from the nearest phone box in floods of tears; he came straight home, armed with flowers, took her in his arms and reassured her as she wept on his shoulders, "we'll get through this," he said, "we'll find a way."

Emily was so grateful for Peter's love and his optimism. Together they agreed that she should at least try and finish medical school. Once again, she felt too guilty to tell him the truth. She alone knew that this time it really was her fault that she had just sabotaged her future career because she couldn't wait to have a baby.

The GP offered Emily an abortion, warning her of the difficulties she would face by continuing the pregnancy. Emily was offended by his attitude, but he was right about difficult. She had to summon every ounce of strength to cope with the nausea which was present twenty-four hours a day and continued throughout the pregnancy. But whether uncomfortable or tired, Emily felt she had no right to complain.

Although Emily loved Peter, she had never learnt to trust anyone enough to share her innermost feelings. Boarding school had taught her how to be an island, and Peter had no idea of what was really going on inside her head. The saving grace in the situation was that Emily's anxiety about the future was balanced by the genuine joy she felt at the prospect of having a baby.

While Emily drove herself hard, nothing less was expected of her in the medical world. During their obstetrics placement, medical students were mandated to deliver a minimum of ten babies, which placed them in direct competition with the student midwives. There was an unwritten rule that if the medical students wanted to deliver babies, they had better not keep the midwives waiting when called to labour ward, day or night to stitch up the unfortunate women who were routinely given episiotomies during childbirth.

Jess was a midwife, radical in her day and spoke passionately against the harms of unnecessary interventions during labour and childbirth, denouncing the practice of routine episiotomies. Emily heard her lecture and was very relieved when she agreed to deliver the baby.

## PLANNING

Peter and Emily did their best to plan for the future. They applied for a one hundred per cent mortgage and looked for affordable properties in the vicinity of the church, which was still the focus of their community. The choice in their price range was extremely limited, but undeterred they made an offer on a maisonette in need of complete renovation. Peter and Emily were delighted when their application for a grant for essential improvements was also accepted by Lambeth Council. The property needed replumbing, rewiring, and the installation of a heating system as well as a kitchen.

The church was organising a summer holiday together. Edward was now a qualified doctor working in paediatrics and was married to Laura. She had been part of a new, radical branch of Christianity known as the 'house-church' movement who claimed to be even more authentic than the charismatics at the Baptist church. Laura was also in the last few months of pregnancy and had been asked to lead the worship for the church holiday. She started a little music group, asking Peter to play keyboard and also invited two other couples who were also expecting their first babies. It was a welcome distraction for Emily, and she soon became friends with the other pregnant women. Admittedly she was envious that they were all on maternity leave and had no plans to return to work once their babies were born.

Laura's previous house-church leaders had been invited to do some bible teaching on the holiday and despite their relative youth, they were fervent about their faith. Unlike traditional church ministers, they had no formal theological training, yet their enthusiasm was contagious, and they seemed very knowledgeable. After the holiday, Edward called a meeting to announce that he and Laura were leaving the Baptist church to start a new house-church supported by these leaders. Emily felt excited when she and Peter were invited to join this very close-knit group of young people who appeared so dedicated and caring towards each other.

## EXPECTING

Back at medical school, with only a couple of weeks left of her final surgical attachment, quite unexpectedly, an empty cot appeared in the middle of the adult ward. The consultant came in for his ward round, turned to the medical students and said, "I can see we are prepared for all eventualities!"

Emily laughed. But it was a stark reminder that the medical school hierarchy had paid little attention to the fact that she was in an advanced state of pregnancy. As medical students they were all expected to assist during operations and the women's theatre scrubs no longer fitted Emily now she was near to term. It was embarrassing having to borrow from the male changing rooms. On the final day of her surgical attachment, thirty-eight weeks pregnant and assisting with an operation, she went into labour. Their baby girl was born early the following morning and just as she expected, Emily fell in love with her immediately.

## LOVE AT FIRST SIGHT

Perhaps it's regrettable that Emily let everyone think that their firstborn child was the result of an 'accidental' pregnancy, when the reality was that Emily's baby girl was very much wanted and hardly an accident. But it didn't change the reality that Peter and

Emily were both over the moon. It changed everything; Emily didn't care about being a doctor anymore, she just wanted to be at home, but something pushed her forwards and she sat the written finals two weeks after Rachel was born. There was a short holiday timetabled before the medical students were due to go away for their three-month elective, which Emily had arranged to do locally in a hospice. But fate intervened when Professor June Lloyd, the new dean of the medical school and a paediatrician, summoned Emily to her office. Emily had failed two of the four papers and Professor Lloyd was frank with her opinion. She told Emily that caring for a newborn baby was far more valuable to her medical training than any three-month elective and so she reassigned Emily to spend the time at home, ostensibly preparing to resit the two exams she had failed. This was such a welcome respite and filled Emily with the courage she needed to finish her medical school training. She passed the resits and then there was only another four months before the June finals and if successful, Emily would leave medical school, qualified as a doctor.

## REPERCUSSIONS

Peter and Emily hadn't anticipated that leaving the Baptist church would upset their friends so much. They were surprised when the kind offer of childcare was withdrawn. Then they were struck with another blow as Lambeth Council went on strike before they had the required permissions to start the essential renovation work on their new flat, and it still wasn't habitable. Without the council's approval, they would lose the valuable grant altogether. Despairing at the double catastrophe, Peter and Emily shared their dilemmas with their new house-church friends. It was Edward and Laura who offered a solution.

Laura's own baby was just a few weeks older than baby Rachel and she offered to look after her just until Emily finished medical school. The winter was cold, and they were still living in the rented house; there was ice on the inside of the windows. So when Edward and Laura suggested it would be easier for everyone if they came to live with them in their lovely, big, centrally heated house with a proper bathroom and inside toilets, it seemed like an answer to prayer. Peter and Emily were incredibly grateful.

Edward, who was now both their landlord and their church leader, was doing research into childhood allergies when baby Rachel developed severe eczema. Eagerly he recruited Rachel into his trial and referred her to a dermatologist. Emily had planned to stop breastfeeding in time for the last four months of medical school, but now she was advised to exclusively breastfeed Rachel until she was six months old and instructed not to give her any cow's milk until after her first birthday. There were no other breast milk substitutes available at the time, so it was hard going when Emily found herself having to express milk in the middle of the night as well as give Rachel night-time feeds, to make sure there was an adequate supply for the next day. Of course, Emily felt she was in no position to complain with all the kindness being shown to her.

However, the biggest struggle for Emily was in leaving baby Rachel at all, so she always rushed back as early as she could after her medical school day was over. By the time the June exams came round, Emily was exhausted. Somehow she passed her finals but now as a qualified doctor, she knew there was no way she could do her pre-registration housejobs. Colleagues warned her that if she gave up now, it was tantamount to career suicide, but Emily wasn't overly concerned. She thought it would work out somehow; it had so far, after all, God was in control.

* * *

*Emily's ability to deceive herself as well as others was firmly entrenched, having learnt to bury her emotions and keep quiet about her difficulties. It was not something she was aware of at that time. Do you think you may be withholding your feelings from those closest to you? Sometimes it is worth finding an outside, independent person like a peer supporter who can listen without judgement.*

# CHAPTER 8

# Life with young children

The Lambeth Council strike carried on, so Peter and Emily made the difficult decision to forfeit the grant and cover the costs of renovation. They did as much work as they could themselves and once the maisonette was habitable, they took in a lodger to help pay the bills. A year later, Jess attended Emily for a home birth and Steve was born; now they were a family of four.

## CHRISTIAN WIVES

The new house-church was not doing too well. Peter and Emily felt uncomfortable when the leaders pried into their private lives under the auspices of pastoral care. Even when the church merged with another whose leadership seemed more experienced, the dogma hardly changed. They were particularly heavy-handed as they taught on scriptures which they said stipulated that the husband was the head of the household and once married, the wife's main duty was to bring up children. It wasn't difficult for Emily to accept her role as a housewife, she enjoyed being at home and had voluntarily relinquished her medical career, but as a couple, Peter and Emily didn't fit the required mould.

One Sunday, some leaders from a related church came to preach. Emily noticed how the rule which prohibited women from speaking in church didn't seem to apply to the leaders' wives and this occasion proved to be no exception. The wife delivered a 'prophetic word'; she said that God had shown her that there was a woman in the room who was not submitted to her husband and as a result, her husband was unable to be the person God meant him to be. Emily froze. It had to be her. God had read her mind and had seen how she tried to push Peter to be more extrovert in his role as head of the household. The leaders prayed for her and from then on Emily did her utmost to become quiet and non-contentious and make herself into a submissive wife.

## EXPANSIVE PLANS

After their third baby Natalie was born, also at home with Jess in attendance, Peter and Emily thought seriously about going overseas. Peter was not enamoured with his career as a computer programmer and Emily longed to return to South-East Asia.

Peter was surprised to be successful when he applied to be Thailand director for a charity called Christian Outreach, an NGO providing aid to refugees and displaced persons on the Thai-Kampuchean border. Emily was given a notional title as medical adviser to the team of volunteers who worked with Christian Outreach. None of them were salaried, but all their expenses were paid, and Emily was excited as they packed up their home, in preparation for the move to Bangkok.

They arrived in April 1987 in the middle of the hot season and as they stepped off the plane, it felt like being hit by a wall of heat. The family were collected from the airport in the Christian Outreach vehicle. Peter and Emily, with their three children under the age of five, sat in the back of a pickup truck, on their way to a new home. The flat was on the seventh floor and a spark flew out as Emily attempted to switch on the ceiling fan. Peter, in particular, demonstrated an incredible degree of versatility, as he adapted to a very different way of life in an extremely hot and humid climate in a totally unfamiliar culture.

## CHARITY WORK

Most of the Christian Outreach team were based in the town of Aranyaprathet, close to the camps of 'displaced people' on the border with Cambodia. Peter's office, the central hub for administration was in Bangkok, but he visited the border every fortnight. Peter positively thrived in his role. He was an excellent administrator, and well able to manage the budgets he controlled. He was just the right temperament to work in Thailand, quietly spoken, polite, yet firm in his views. His persistent determination lent weight as he managed the politics, advocating for the displaced Cambodians. Peter became a vital member at the monthly meeting in Bangkok when the directors of the NGOs who ran the border relief operations, met with Thai government officials to discuss matters of concern. They appreciated just how well Peter handled these matters. Some had learnt the hard way that loud voices and demanding attitudes were counter-productive, in a culture where it is incredibly important to honour all concerned and not cause loss of face.

In Bangkok, Peter also managed the other side of their charity's work, providing aid to a government-run children's home. Long term, he knew that this work had to be owned by the Thai people and just as he was drafting an advertisement to recruit permanent and suitably qualified local staff, a Thai couple arrived at his office offering their services. A few years later, they set up their own foundation which became the foremost organisation in Thailand, providing support to disabled children and their families. They were instrumental in changing Thai society's views on disability, so that far fewer children were abandoned into care.

## PRISON

Suffice to say, most of Emily's time was spent looking after her own three children, but one day she was visited by the director of an NGO that ran a feeding programme for prisoners detained in the immigration detention centre. They were particularly concerned about a prisoner in one of the packed communal cells. He was emaciated, coughing and desperately ill, clearly in need of medical treatment. Suspecting TB, which had the potential to infect his fellow inmates, they asked for Emily's help. She agreed he looked very sick and naively they smuggled a specimen of his sputum out to be tested. When the result confirmed their fears, they hoped it might persuade the governor of the detention centre to send him to hospital for treatment. But they hadn't read the situation correctly and the resultant loss of face was a serious blunder.

On each daily visit to feed the prisoners, the NGO volunteers were required to surrender their passports. Emily's title of 'Dr' was clear from her passport. When the bell signalled that it was time to leave, Emily was separated from the others and locked inside the jail. They released her a few hours later but it was a terrifying reminder not to fall foul of the rules again. The infected prisoner was released without treatment, near the border with his home country of Myanmar. It is highly unlikely that he survived without access to medical care.

## PRIMARY-SCHOOL PROBLEM

Four-year-old Rachel was enrolled at the same school Emily had attended as a child. At first, she loved it and then for no discernible reason, her behaviour changed. Emily knew something was wrong; it was so unlike their sunny little daughter to be so quiet and withdrawn. When questioned, Rachel's teacher described her as 'very naughty, always hiding in the toilet'. In Thailand, parents were not permitted to enter the premises during school hours and so it was fortuitous when one of the mothers defied the regulation, eager to get a forgotten item to her child. She warned Emily that she wouldn't like what she was going to hear. As this mother crossed the playground, she came across a group of older children and there in the middle was little Rachel, her face puce while one of them had their hands around her neck.

Peter and Emily went straight to the headteacher, but he refused to believe the story or acknowledge this shocking instance of bullying. So, Peter and Emily had little choice and they removed Rachel from the school immediately. Emily decided to home-school Rachel and within a short space of time, she was back to her normal happy self.

## POSTNATAL STRUGGLE

Emily loved looking after her young children but when their fourth baby, Harry, was born, she struggled to cope. The labour had been just one hour long, the birth itself was very rapid, and Emily haemorrhaged. When she was discharged from hospital, it was hard to keep up with the home-schooling, while simultaneously looking after her newborn and attending to the needs of her other two children. Steve was four by this stage and Emily knew she should start teaching him as well. Her courage failed and so reluctantly Peter and Emily agreed that it would be better to return to the UK once the initial two-year period of Peter's contract was over.

A couple of months later, Emily felt much better and regretted that she had instigated their return to the UK. Peter loved his job, and the children had such a great life, swimming every day. Rachel was excelling in her schoolwork and loved her ballet classes, Steve excelled at diving even at age four, and loved playing short tennis, little Natalie learnt to swim around the same time she learnt to walk. All of them had plenty of contact with other children who lived in the same compound as they did. Realising it was a mistake to leave Thailand, they tried to get the decision reversed, but it was too late; Peter's successor had already been appointed. However, Peter was optimistic, sure that he would find further opportunities to work in the charity sector back in the UK.

## MOVE TO SOUTHAMPTON

In April 1989, they returned to England, moving to an ex-council house on the edge of a small green in Southampton. A beautiful magnolia tree was in flower in the back garden. It didn't seem so bad after all. But despite Peter's considerable achievements while running the NGO in Thailand, apparently it carried little weight back in the UK. Eventually he found a job in IT, but Emily knew it wouldn't be fulfilling after his interesting but short-lived career in relief work and she blamed herself for jeopardising his future.

They joined a large and well-established church in Southampton, confident that this time the culture wouldn't be oppressive. It seemed ideal because the church ran its own primary school and after the experience in Bangkok, Emily was keen to protect the children from bullying. She began to feel better about being back, once she started to make friends with parents who had children of similar ages.

A year later, Emily sat on Natalie's tiny bed beneath the window, opposite the bunks where Rachel and Steve slept, she surveyed the overflowing cupboard and her attempts to tidy the toys into a box. One-year-old Harry slept in a cot in the even smaller box room, but it was obvious that the family were rapidly outgrowing the house.

## UPSIZING

Emily couldn't help herself looking at the 'for sale' signs in the locality. She had seen a good-sized property for sale on a main road a couple of miles away. She phoned the estate agent and they sent her the details. Even though she knew it was outside their price range, it seemed ideal, so she arranged a viewing. It was even bigger inside than it had seemed from the outside, perfect but unaffordable. A few weeks later, the estate agent phoned to let them know the owners had dropped the price. The property was empty when they returned for a second look. They stood in the back garden with the agent and Emily voiced her thoughts. "It's perfect. If only they would take..." and she named the price.

The agent replied that the vendors would accept and were so keen to facilitate a quick sale, they would buy Peter and Emily's house at its market value.

It was wonderful to move to a house which was plenty big enough for their family of growing children and the school transport left from a bus stop just down the road. Life was working out but for one thing, as Emily feared – Peter was not happy with his job back in IT. Emily consoled herself that despite her failings, God, who she saw as her benevolent overseer had managed to steer their course so far. She prayed that once again something might fall into place. Nonetheless, she wasn't complacent.

## MAD IDEAS

After supper, when the children were in bed, Peter and Emily snuggled up on the sofa together in a rare moment of quiet. Emily decided to share her mad idea of how she was wondering if there might be some way of doing her pre-registration year part-time. If she then went on to become a GP, their future would be secure, and Peter could do something more fulfilling. Peter thought there was no harm in finding out.

There was no official pathway to enable any doctor to work the mandatory pre-registration year part-time. Women were still a significant minority at medical school, and it was unusual to graduate with a baby or young children. Even though it was over seven years since she had qualified as a doctor, in the autumn of 1990, she wrote to the local postgraduate dean asking if they knew of anyone who might want to job-share with her.

The response was exciting. A single parent was due to qualify in the summer of 1991 and also wanted to work part-time. Emily needed to get her documentation sorted; she wrote to St George's Medical School asking for references and also arranged to meet Leah. Meanwhile, she scanned the weekly job advertisements in the *British Medical Journal (BMJ)*.

She was slightly startled when she saw that an urgent vacancy had arisen for a six-month pre-registration surgical house officer post in Basingstoke, due to start on 1st February 1991. Knowing that the earliest potential job share couldn't start before August, Emily mooted the idea of a role swap with Peter, "just to work full-time for six months," she said.

## INTERVIEW

It was extremely nerve-wracking when Emily was called for interview. The two candidates sat waiting on upholstered chairs in the corridor outside the doctors' mess. The consultant surgeons called Emily in first and after what seemed like a barrage of questions, she was asked to wait outside. It seemed an eternity, sitting there trying to predict her chances, while they interviewed the other candidate. Then she was summoned back into the room, only to be told that they were not going to offer her the job. One of the consultants spelt it out, "it is highly unlikely that anyone will employ you, given the time that has elapsed since you finished medical school. Have you thought about what else you're going to do?"

It felt like a red rag to a bull, and Emily was defiant. "There are two kinds of people when thrown into deep water, those who sink and those who swim, and I am going to swim!"

They asked her to wait outside again and she sat bemused and trembling after her outburst, nursing her disappointment, and wondering why she couldn't just go home. When they called her in for a third time, the surgeons told Emily that her final answer had changed their minds – she had the job.

Before Emily started at Basingstoke, she met Leah, the medical student who wanted to work part-time; they agreed to make a joint application to job-share, working half-time for a year to complete the six-month equivalent medical house job from August 1991 – August 1992. They were successful and it was thought to be the first ever job-share in Britain for pre-registration house-officer posts.

* * *

*People who end up with emotional or psychological problems are often thought of as being less resilient than most. Everyone's situation must be considered within the context of the rest of their lives. What worked in the past may not help in the future. Are you someone whose attributes are not fully appreciated, or whose achievements are undermined because of your current state of health or circumstances?*

# CHAPTER 9

# Working as a doctor

Emily had enjoyed being a housewife and was proud of the way she catered for her family's needs. It was hard to let go as she prepared to hand it over to Peter for the role-swap. When she had any time to herself during the preceding few weeks, Emily had genned up on the subject of general surgery as best she could, reading textbooks and revising from her old lecture notes. She only had a couple of days to shadow the existing surgical house officer, and then on her first day as a doctor, there she was holding a bleep, on call. Near to midnight, she finally made it to bed in the tiny on-call room located just off the surgical wards, but it wasn't long before she was disturbed. She was summoned to A&E, to assist the senior registrar (SR).

It was a shock to discover that a man had been brought in by ambulance with a gunshot wound to his chest; the SR had tried to perform life-saving surgery right there in A&E. He died. Shortly afterwards, paramedics wheeled another patient into the resuscitation room. This man had been stabbed in a completely unrelated incident and was also critically ill and unresponsive. Emily was astounded to find herself assisting as the SR first cut open the patient's abdomen and then his chest. It all happened so fast, but this surgery was also unsuccessful, and the patient died.

## SETTLING IN

Emily returned to the on-call room and sat on the bed. She tried not to freak out as her mind replayed what she had just witnessed. It transpired that the events of the night were incredibly rare and she didn't have to attend to any further incidents of violent assault for many years to come.

After the first week or so, Emily's nerves settled, and she found her feet. Determined not to let the consultants down when they had clearly taken a risk in employing her, Emily aspired to excellence. She became accustomed to the uninvited commentary about her age and status as a mother. "This has got to be better than washing nappies all day, eh?" Mr Ray, one of the consultants, would say as he asked her to do something particularly unsavoury in the operating theatre. Emily laughed with the jokes although it was wearing. She knew that she needed to perform over and above her younger peer group, just to prove that she was good at her job.

Emily adapted quickly, learning to compartmentalise her life. But during the hour's drive home, she had to consciously switch back into her role as Mum. She felt slightly guilty that she enjoyed her job and also at leaving the children, but it was some consolation knowing that they didn't appear to miss her. Peter also appeared to be happy and thriving, having developed his own way of running the household. Occasionally Emily wished she didn't feel quite so redundant at home.

It was hard to be away for a night on call or a whole weekend at work, from early Saturday morning to Monday evening and she landed with a guilt trip. As a result, however tired she was, Emily tried to make up for it and insisted on joining in with as many family activities as possible. On Saturday mornings she went swimming with the children, she watched Steve doing football or accompanied the girls to their dance classes. When threatened with overwhelming fatigue, Emily reminded herself that she had made it through medical school. She laughed off the nights on call, equating them to the years of disturbed nights when the babies were small.

In retrospect it seems ridiculous how little attention Emily paid to her own welfare. But this was nothing unusual in the medical culture of the nineties, when personal well-being, healthy life-work balance and self-care were never part of the conversation. Complaints about such things were a sign of weakness and doctors saw it as a matter of pride to push oneself to the limit. To be fair, none of Emily's non-medical friends or family had any more concern than she did.

## VALIDATION

In July, as the end of the six months approached, the two consultants invited both Emily and Peter up to Basingstoke for dinner and paid for their stay in a hotel. They were extraordinarily generous and presented Emily with a cheque, saying that quite contrary to their expectations, she had been the best junior doctor they had ever had. Emily was exhilarated; she had redeemed herself and revelled in the kind of affirmation that she had craved all through her life.

The experience of working as a surgical house officer was useful when she met with Leah to plan how to make their job-share work. It was important for everyone that they devise a seamless way of sharing the workload to minimise any disruption to patient care. They decided that they would both work full-time but on alternate weeks, with a comprehensive handover to one another on Wednesday mornings. It was very successful, and the consultants were impressed.

## MONEY WORRY

Emily was only being paid half a house-officer salary and it was not enough to support the household. Peter had also planned to work part-time, but it became very difficult since there always had to be someone available to look after two-year-old Harry, as well as all four of the children after school. Peter's business did not thrive under the restrictions imposed by their circumstances. They reviewed their situation and concluded it would be better if Emily worked additional hours during her 'week off'. There were plenty of locum vacancies in the Royal South Hants Hospital where she was based. They also decided that she would become full-time again after the job-share ended, hopeful that it would only take another three years to become a GP. Then she would have no difficulty working part-time and would be earning a decent salary. It seemed a win-win to have Peter back as a full-time Dad which gave the children a guaranteed stability as they grew up.

## CULTURES

Junior doctors such as Emily were expected to be dedicated to long hours, and the hospital provided a 'mess' where they could make hot drinks or watch TV while they had a break. It wasn't the most salubrious of facilities, and the brown covers on the sofas were worn and stained. But it was some respite from the mêlée and somewhere to gather and chat with white-coated colleagues, even though it was annoying to be disturbed by the frequent high-pitched sounds of the bleep going off, particularly just as a film got going on the TV.

Emily was in the minority amongst the junior doctors, most of whom were men. More so for being a mother, when most female doctors delayed starting a family until they were on less onerous rotas or working in jobs with more sociable hours.

Medicine was still steeped in hierarchy and patriarchy, but so was the church where Emily was a member. The leaders were much revered and respected, considered wise, almost as if bestowed with special knowledge that the rest of the church did not have. Many of the six-hundred-strong membership were professionals themselves – doctors, teachers, nurses, solicitors. Furthermore, the church was suspicious of 'non-Christians', unable to countenance that 'unbelievers' could have as much wisdom or insight as they did.

Emily lived in the same area as some of the church leaders. Their children played together and went to the same school. As a couple, Peter and Emily sometimes felt excluded from the close-knit inner circle of friendship in their locality, but they had every reason to trust the leaders.

Naturally, Emily struggled with fatigue, but frequently reminded herself how she had managed so far. Boarding school had taught her well – there was nothing to be gained by complaining and she coped with stress by working even harder. When at home, Emily deferred her own needs while she tried her best to be a good mother to the children who she missed so much during her long working hours. But it was all getting a bit much.

## SUPERWOMAN FLAGGING

One Saturday morning, Emily arranged to visit one of the church elders who lived in their neighbourhood. She sat in the front room looking out on the tall beech trees in the front garden. Joan was a warm-hearted Scottish lady with white curly hair, about the same age as Emily's mother. She gave Emily a hug and held her hand while she poured out her heart, describing how hard she was finding it to combine work with family life. Joan patted her leg sympathetically. "Let's pray, Emily, the Lord will give you all the strength you need."

## A&E

In August 1992, Emily progressed to the next stage in a junior doctor's life. If she was to become a GP, she would need to work a series of four more six-month hospital posts, now in the 'senior house officer' (SHO) grade. She started the first of these in A&E at Southampton General Hospital. It was good because the SHOs worked a full-shift system which reduced the overall number of hours to seventy per week, and it suited family life better. When she worked a full week of nights, it would be followed by a whole week off; it felt such a treat to be able to enjoy time off, without the pressure to supplement her income by working additional hours.

## AFTER SCHOOL

Between them, the children had many after-school activities. Both of the little girls loved their dance classes, and the boys were equally focused on their sports, particularly football. However, not long after they arrived back from Thailand, Rachel's ballet teacher spotted her talents. When she suggested that Rachel take up additional classes and enter for dance exams, Emily wasn't keen. She wanted Rachel's dance lessons to be fun and didn't want her to feel pressurised. But she needn't have worried because Rachel's appetite seemed insatiable, and she constantly asked to do more. By the time she was seven, her teacher suggested she audition for the monthly junior associate class at the Royal Ballet School in London.

## JUNIOR ASSOCIATES

Rachel was successful and Emily was very much in awe as they walked through the wood-panelled corridors of the famous Royal Ballet School. The walls were adorned with photos of famous dancers and the pleasant aroma of polish embellished the school's indefinable atmosphere; this was a place where history was made, where some of the most famous ballet dancers of all time, such as Margot Fonteyn and Rudolf Nureyev, had rehearsed, and dancers of the future were trained.

Many of the parents travelled some distance to bring their young children to the special monthly junior associate class and, like Emily, sat in the canteen until their child's class had finished. Senior students from the Royal Ballet School came and went during their breaks in classes or rehearsals, pianos tinkling away in the background. It felt surreal. Emily was mindful of her own childhood dreams and was well aware that she must not try and live them out through her daughter. She knew that her priority was to support Rachel, and she must never be the driving force behind her future. While Emily tried to stay both neutral and realistic, Rachel loved every minute of her classes; there was no doubt that she possessed her own intrinsic motivation to succeed.

When Rachel was eight, one of her friends from Southampton also joined her for the junior associate classes; that made life easier for Peter and Emily, as now they could share the monthly drive to London with another family. It became clear that the junior associate classes were part of the Royal Ballet School's attempt to cast their net wide as they sought talented children for admission to White Lodge, the Royal Ballet Junior School. They took students from the age of eleven and competition was fierce with applicants from all over the world.

Rachel remained keen to apply for a place, but it presented Emily with an enormous dilemma. If successful, then Rachel would have to board during the week, and Emily had sworn to herself, and then to Peter, that she would never let any of her children go to boarding school after her own miserable experiences. At first, these considerations seemed a little wild as the junior associates' teacher constantly reminded both the children and their parents not to get their hopes up high. The selection process was rigorous, and very few children would be successful. Reassured, Emily was able to brush off her anxieties and take life one step at a time.

## MEDICAL MAYHEM

After six months in A&E, Emily moved on to do two more SHO posts that would also count towards her future career as a GP. First was obstetrics and gynaecology followed by six months of paediatrics.

At the start of paediatrics, the consultant reassured Emily that he was always there to give assistance if needed. As soon as she arrived for her first day carrying the on-call bleep for paediatrics, she was called to the labour ward. The midwife handed Emily a pale, floppy, unresponsive baby, who was making no attempt to breathe. Knowing she was out of her depth and needed the consultant's help, Emily put out a fast bleep – the signal that this was an emergency – to summon the consultant immediately. She was far too inexperienced to resuscitate a critically ill baby on her own, but Emily had no choice. As she inflated the baby's lungs with a bag and mask, she desperately hoped the baby would start breathing on her own. The obstetric registrar came over to help and as the baby's heart rate slowed, they started CPR. There was no sign of the consultant and Emily began to panic. She yelled as loudly as she could, "Just get some help."

A consultant anaesthetist responded to the call and placed a tube in the baby's trachea to control her breathing. The anaesthetist didn't know the correct dose of adrenalin for a baby, and nor it seemed, did anyone else. Usually the doses were easy to find, printed out as an aide memoire, but on that fateful day someone had taken it off the wall in order to get the sheet laminated. Emily was panic-stricken as she tried to remember how to calculate the dose. As the anaesthetist gave the adrenalin, the baby's heartbeat increased, her colour improved and at last she started to breathe on her own. Just at that moment, the consultant paediatrician burst through the door. He explained that he confused the 'fast bleep', to summon him urgently, with the 'test bleep', which always took place at that time.

But Emily was too distracted by her own horrifying realisation that she had miscalculated the dose of adrenalin and immediately confessed to her boss, the paediatrician. He wasn't worried. "Look at the baby," he said. "She's fine. You saved her life."

The consultant was right of course, but Emily couldn't see it that way. The incident played over and over in her mind and every time she thought about it, she felt as though she couldn't breathe.

The system had failed, leaving inexperienced junior doctors to deal with a life-threatening emergency. Even though there had been two other doctors present who were more senior than she was, the consultant who promised he'd always be available had not arrived, when Emily called for help. Even though the baby was fine, Emily couldn't process the experience logically. All she could think about was the fact that she had difficulty remembering the exact dose of adrenalin. There was no debrief and no further discussion.

Undoubtedly it was a very difficult situation for all concerned and Emily felt terrible as she wondered how the baby's poor mother coped during the whole fiasco. But her own vulnerability manifested itself, both as repeated self-castigation and as terror that she might make a fatal mistake in future.

INJURY

At the weekend Emily was injured while playing with the children on the flume at the local swimming pool. She was admitted to hospital for an emergency operation and then while recovering at home, she developed sciatica down both her legs. Her run of ill health didn't stop when this was followed by severe diarrhoea and she became unwell, losing weight. She was readmitted to hospital under a gastro-enterologist who was convinced she had an underlying cancer and subjected her to a battery of unpleasant investigations. When the tests all came back as normal, his attitude changed. At first, Emily couldn't grasp what he was saying and then the penny dropped; she felt both embarrassed and humiliated at the thought that she had wasted everyone's time, never mind what she had been through.

Her GP read out the gastro-enterologist's letter stating that her illness was purely psychosomatic. Emily felt even more upset, triggered by the memory of school days and the letter from the horrible neurologist who had said she could stop shaking any time she wanted. But she acknowledged that the gastro-enterologist was probably right and her unexplained illness was likely stress-related. However, she still felt very misunderstood. Her symptoms had been real, unpleasant and the tests had been awful, and now she was being treated as though it was all her own fault.

Knowing that the medical profession saw psychosomatic illness as a sign of weakness, Emily felt angry with herself for allowing it to happen. She defaulted back to her old ways of coping and that meant she just needed to force herself back to work and prove that she was no weakling. But internally, Emily felt confused and upset; what she really wanted to do was collapse in a heap and give up.

\* \* \*

*As humans we are very complex, and the mind can never be separated from the physical body. Sometimes the stress of life, of relationships, of circumstances, or of the past, manifests itself in a physical way. Have you ever had a tension headache or felt sick with anxiety?*

PART 2

# Captive to the toxic cure

# CHAPTER 10

# Dilemma

The whole of Emily's extended family arranged to go on a Christmas holiday together which included a visit to one of the Philippines islands. It was a great opportunity to spend some time away from work with the whole family.

In the spring of 1994, Rachel was still as keen as ever to try for a place at White Lodge, the junior section of the Royal Ballet School. Despite Emily's worries, she sent the requested photos of Rachel in her leotard for the first stage in the application process. Peter and Emily kept Rachel's hopes grounded, knowing full well that the chances of success for each of the numerous applicants from all over the world was slim. During each successive step, children would be eliminated from the group of hopefuls right up until the day of the final auditions. Emily tried hard not to worry about the consequences in the event that Rachel was successful.

## TRAINEE GP

The next changeover date for Emily's job was February 1st 1994, and she arranged to do six months as a trainee GP, hoping for some respite from the stress of the recent hospital posts. She was attached to a practice which served a large council estate, and Emily was expected to play a full part in the on-call rota. She didn't enjoy having to drive herself to patients' homes in the middle of the night, especially when carrying a doctor's bag full of emergency drugs, past the paraphernalia of addiction, as she climbed the stairs of a local tower block. Suddenly the prospect of becoming a GP seemed less attractive.

## AUDITION

Undoubtedly Peter and Emily felt proud of their eleven-year-old daughter when the letter came inviting her to the final auditions at White Lodge. But Emily's ambivalence was huge as she felt caught between the desire to support her daughter's dreams and terrified of the fact that she would be a weekly boarder.

On the big day, all three of them drove to White Lodge, situated in the middle of Richmond Park. All the candidate children were led away to various studios, and the parents were shown to a large room with chairs lining the walls, left to wait it out together. There was little to distract them, despite the incredible architecture and history associated with this famous school. The tension was palpable, especially at distinct points throughout the day, when tearful boys and girls were returned to their parents and the families left with dour faces, as the group dwindled in size. Conversations were muted and the atmosphere could be cut with a knife while the parents knew that the future of their children was being decided behind closed doors, all of them in competition with one another.

As the day passed, it became apparent that Rachel was one of the girls left in the final group. Suddenly she burst through the door beaming, Peter and Emily threw their arms around her, absolutely delighted. Rachel had just won a government-assisted place to the most prestigious ballet school in the world and even Emily was able to celebrate their talented little daughter's success.

## PREPARATION

The summer holidays were a time of great excitement for Rachel as preparations were made for her to start at White Lodge in September. Emily gave herself a stiff talking to, determined to put her reservations aside. Rachel would be coming home every weekend and as parents they were clear – if she didn't like it or changed her mind, they would never force her to stay.

The Royal Ballet School was the feeder for the company, and they only took children who they thought had the greatest potential to become professional dancers in the future. Peter and Emily had little doubt that this was a tough call, but they had no idea what it would really be like for their daughter. Every student had their place guaranteed only for a year at a time, with a major reassessment every summer. It was an incredible pressure – it wasn't just Rachel's talent that was under scrutiny but also the way her body developed through adolescence. Even if she continued to be successful, all ballet dancers were forever plagued by the risk of injury. But at that moment, Emily's major concern was the intrusive memories of her own boarding school experiences.

## CRISIS

In August, Emily was in the throes of crisis, she made an appointment with one of the partners at her GP practice; all the doctors there were Christians and most were part of her own church community. Perhaps the boundaries were blurred. Sitting in the modern waiting room, too nervous to even look at the magazines, Emily rehearsed how she was going to explain her insomnia and exhaustion. She was hoping for sympathy, but the GP thought she was depressed and prescribed Prozac (fluoxetine). Emily wished she had been given longer to talk about what was bothering her, because what she really wanted was to feel understood and for the merry-go-round of her life to stop, rather than be given pills to swallow. However, she didn't object as she left the consultation room, prescription in her hand, exhibiting her well-established pattern of deference to authority figures. Emily took the concrete stairs down to the car park, barely able to think.

Perhaps the GP was short of time that day. Perhaps if the GP had really heard what Emily was trying to say, she would have handled it differently. Perhaps she might have said, "You've had a very stressful time, especially working such gruelling hours as a junior doctor and you're dealing with the recently triggered, painful memories of boarding school. No wonder you're feeling low and exhausted. Why don't you talk to the practice counsellor? You need some time to recuperate."

Emily really didn't think she was depressed, and she didn't want to take medication. But after her recent psychosomatic illness, reluctantly she thought she had better give Prozac a try. When it made her feel both sick and restless, she decided not to renew the prescription.

## LYMINGTON

Emily had already started at her last hospital post which would contribute to the completion of her training as a GP. This time, although it was another A&E job, she would be working both at the small casualty department in Lymington and the main department in Southampton. Gordon Walker, the lead consultant, thought Emily was ideal because she already had six months' experience of A&E. He reassured her that Lymington casualty would be very quiet when she was the only doctor on duty during the nights and weekends when she would be resident on call.

The new A&E consultant, Liz Cleverly, was inspiring and an excellent teacher. Emily was delighted when for the very first time as a junior doctor she received formal training in resuscitation and the treatment of severely injured patients. It was Liz who drew Emily's attention to an innovative scheme which had just been launched to support doctors to continue their postgraduate training part-time. Recognising Emily's enthusiasm, she encouraged Emily to apply to train to become a consultant in emergency medicine. The scheme made it possible for Emily to work part-time on a viable salary and she was due to start on 1st February 1995.

Rachel started her first term at White Lodge just before her twelfth birthday. Every weekend she came home enthusing about it and Emily realised she needn't have worried. Life was looking up, even though the childhood memories were still very active in her mind.

## ANOTHER PAEDIATRIC EMERGENCY

The weather was still warm on a Saturday afternoon in late September when Emily was working the weekend in Lymington Casualty. Without prior warning, wailing sirens and blue flashing lights declared the arrival of an emergency ambulance. Paramedics rushed inside with a very young child, hastily explaining he had been found beside a bouncy castle. CPR was already in progress and Emily swung into action, glad of Liz's teaching as she led the ongoing resuscitation. She did everything she possibly could to try and save the little boy's life but he never regained consciousness, and he died. The experienced nursing sister accompanied Emily to give the devastating news to his parents, who had arrived in their own transport. They had thought that their child had been perfectly healthy before this tragic afternoon. All anyone could do was wait for the results of the post-mortem.

The parents returned the following day and asked Emily if she would accompany them to the chapel of rest to spend some more time with their child's little body. They placed a favourite toy beside the tiny, shrouded figure and asked everyone to join hands while they sang a favourite song. It broke Emily's heart.

Unable to stop herself from identifying with the parents, Emily imagined how she would feel if this was one of her own children. She went over the attempt at resuscitation again and again, wondering if there was anything more that could have been done to save this child.

Later that week, Liz Cleverly scrutinised the case and praised Emily for the way she had handled it, but Emily didn't feel ready for this degree of responsibility. The post-mortem result confirmed that the child had an undiagnosed, life-limiting medical condition. Nothing would have changed the outcome.

Despite this new information, Emily felt worse than ever. It felt very similar to the experience with the newborn baby, and she had nightmares of shouting for help and nobody coming to the rescue. Feeling overwhelmed, Emily lost confidence and felt increasingly anxious every day as she got into her car to drive to work.

At church, Emily asked for prayer. People were kind but gave only superficial entreaties, such as "surrender it all to God" or "the joy of the Lord is your strength". It was no help at all. Emily sought out some of the doctors who also went to the church. They were sympathetic, but invariably reciprocated by telling her about the awful things that had happened to them during their careers. Far from reassuring her, it seemed to Emily that everyone else was able to cope, and she felt alone and ashamed because she so obviously couldn't.

## ANOTHER CRISIS

Following a particularly bad night when she hardly slept, Emily found herself thinking more about the depression diagnosis from a couple of months earlier. Maybe the GP was right. She looked it up in her textbook and sure enough, the symptoms were all there. She was miserable, stressed, couldn't sleep, and had lost her appetite. Close to breaking point, Emily had to do something, and went to find the consultant after work. Unfortunately, Liz wasn't around, so Emily told Gordon she thought she was depressed. "No, you're not, Emily," he responded. "There's nothing wrong with your work."

When Emily broke down in tears it was as if she had thrown down the gauntlet. Gordon didn't suggest that her feelings were normal given the circumstances and he made a referral to the sick doctors' counselling service. Emily didn't know of any other doctor who had been through similar struggles; she felt isolated.

It was December when Emily found herself nervously waiting for another GP appointment. This time the GP looked really concerned when Emily tearfully listed her symptoms. The GP apologised that she had to put 'depression' on the sick note. There had to be a legitimate reason for Emily to be signed off work. She also prescribed a different antidepressant, and then warned Emily that it would take six weeks to be effective, while simultaneously reassuring her that it would help her recover more quickly. This time, Emily was desperate enough to comply.

Neither Emily, nor presumably the GP, knew that the myth of chemical imbalance was pedalled by the pharmaceutical companies. Consequently, doctors prescribed antidepressants to cure a non-existent serotonin deficiency in the brain – and in doing so very successfully caused a neurochemical imbalance not just in the brain, but throughout the body. Emily and her doctor were also ignorant that suddenly stopping psychiatric drugs like Prozac could provoke withdrawal reactions, which might well mimic the very symptoms the drug was supposed to treat.

On the second antidepressant drug, Emily felt numbed out, but it did nothing to extinguish the powerful emotions. She felt utterly miserable, but unable to cry. Internally, the pressure was building, externally, the world felt unreal. Despite the GP's assurance that the side effects would soon pass, and that she would soon start to feel better, Emily felt worse. It was very frightening when she found herself thinking about suicide.

## FULL-BLOWN BREAKDOWN

Emily knew what was behind her breakdown and was grateful that Gordon had referred her for counselling. It was so obviously caused by fatigue, stress due to the recent tragedy at work, and not least the resurgence of memories from boarding school. There was only a couple of months before Emily's flexible (part-time) training in A&E was due to begin, and she hoped that reducing her hours would help the situation.

The appointment with 'The Sick Doctors Counselling Service' took place at the DOP (Department of Psychiatry), part of the Royal South Hants Hospital in Southampton. Emily was assessed by a consultant psychiatrist who was also trained as a psychotherapist, and she sent a letter to the GP outlining the context of Emily's distress, noting many of the triggering factors.

- Working 80-120 hours a week for the better part of five years as the financial provider for the family, in a highly stressful job.
- Experienced several recent, significant, and highly traumatic work-related experiences involving the death or near-death of children.

- Making considerable efforts to maintain her role as mother to four school-age children, often sacrificing her own self-care in the process.
- A resurgence of painful childhood memories from time at boarding school, triggered when her eldest daughter won a place at the Royal Ballet School.
- Little emotional support from her community.

Clearly, Emily needed help but was it coming from the right people in the right place when 'The Sick Doctors Counselling Service' usually took referrals for addicted doctors?

There was no mention that Emily's emotional crisis was reasonable given the circumstances. Emily was told that she would be put on the waiting list for counselling and advised to continue antidepressants. Perhaps what she really needed was validation of her symptoms, and advice that she had overreached her limits. Some empathic guidance on self-care involving her spouse would not have gone amiss. But Emily and Peter were never considered together as a couple, let alone as a family.

When Emily received the appointment for counselling, she had been assigned to a trainee psychiatrist for psychodynamic psychotherapy. Perhaps a more experienced therapist who understood childhood trauma might have helped her realign her embedded, erroneous self-beliefs. Perhaps a different modality would have been better rather than a blank-screen approach of psychodynamic psychotherapy where the therapist withheld facial expression and overt empathy – much like the blank and expressionless mother during the 'still face' experiment with the baby. Instead, Emily was expected to talk about painful memories at a time when she was more than usually stressed and exhausted, while she felt numbed out and very unreal because of antidepressants. Is it any wonder that she didn't feel any better?

## VOICE OF SANITY

Liz Cleverly, her supportive A&E consultant, came to see Emily at home shortly after Christmas. As they sat drinking tea in the sitting room, Liz encouraged Emily to rest until February when she was due to start the new, part-time, flexible training scheme. Regretfully Liz's voice of sanity came too late to prevent Emily's spiral downwards and she never made it back to work.

This was the pivotal point in Emily's life. Although the root causes of her emotional distress had been acknowledged, the emphasis of treatment was aimed at correcting a non-existent chemical imbalance for the psychiatric diagnosis of depression.

\* \* \*

*While a psychiatric diagnosis may bring transient relief through the acknowledgement that something is really wrong, it is important to consider the implications. Have you been given a diagnosis that is helpful? Do you feel understood by your doctor, your therapist, your family, and your community? Have you considered if there are other options?*

# CHAPTER 11

# First admission

The time off sick could have been the perfect opportunity for a much-needed break; a chance to read a favourite John Grisham thriller or a Maeve Binchy without interruption. She no longer had a baby who required feeding or a toddler wanting a drink or the call, "Mummy, I'm finished. Can you come and wipe me?"

## ISOLATION

Instead, Emily banished herself to the bedroom, spending most of her time in self-imposed isolation, where she lay obsessed by haunting memories which she ruminated on all day long. She didn't talk to Peter; she thought she should protect him from her troubles. Left alone with chaotic and confusing thoughts, Emily's symptoms spiralled.

Emily felt irritated by the sky blue of the bedroom walls which somehow never got redecorated. She hated the whiteness of the monstrosity of the wall unit which they hadn't got round to replacing. She stared at the lampshade and resented its tassels, a product of a bygone era, out of date and left by the previous owners. Outside, the winter sky was murky grey through the two sash windows which were ten feet away from similar windows in the neighbour's house. There was nothing to distract her from misery.

Emily forgot she had a sense of humour; she forgot how she and Peter would laugh over the silliest things as they lay in bed together. She lost any joy that could be found either in her memories or in her imagination. Emily couldn't understand how it had come to this and believed she had no right to feel this way. She'd heard the derogatory way colleagues talked about patients who were anxious or depressed. Mental illness was something that happened to other people, not to doctors who want to train in A&E to become consultants. All that existed in Emily's world was predicated by worry about the future and despair about the past. She couldn't see any way through this, fretting that she might f*ck up at work and catastrophising how she would then get struck off the medical register.

In addition to feeling emotionally numb, Emily felt restless and shaky, and couldn't sleep. She had no energy and couldn't get up. Undoubtedly, daytime inactivity compounded the insomnia, and Emily felt worse than ever. She couldn't read, in fact she couldn't do anything, with the exception of her mind, which had taken on a life of its own. This could not be shut down, and it whirred away, round and round, stuck in a cycle of unanswerable questions and irreversible memories. While Emily's attention focused on every wrong turn she had made, she completely lost perspective.

Increasingly distanced from her loving and supportive husband, Emily had decided he would never be able to understand what she was going through. As Emily gave in to despair, she became increasingly helpless and the complete opposite to her usual independent self who pushed through difficulties. What had happened to the fighter, full of determination, aspiring to excellence in her career? Where was the superhero martyred to the cause of supporting her family while working in a difficult job as a junior doctor? On previous occasions, Emily had a good track record of pushing through at times of crisis. But not this time. While the doctors confirmed the diagnosis of depression, they also told her that antidepressant drugs held the answers.

## WORSE ON PROZAC

Although some people feel better when they are taking antidepressants, Emily's symptoms had become progressively worse ever since she started Prozac. While it was known that thoughts of self-harm and suicide could increase when the newer antidepressants (SSRIs) were taken by children and young people, the evidence that some *healthy adult volunteers given these drugs also developed thoughts of self-harm and suicide* had not been made public. It is notable that Emily had absolutely no thoughts of self-harm or suicide *before* she started taking antidepressants.

The short winter days and long sleepless nights repeated in unbearable monotony. "You'll feel better in the spring," said the hopefuls. But Emily felt her life draining away, like bath-water swirling round the plug hole, inevitable, unstoppable, down, down, down into the sewer.

The vulnerable child version of Emily had returned to the fore, without clear boundaries of where she ended, and the rest of the world began. Without fail, the memories which surfaced were not the happy ones. Emily realised her mother had been right when she was a child. "Why would everyone be looking at *you*? You're not the only person around."

Of course, her mother had meant it kindly, trying to discourage Emily from agonising over her goofy teeth, but instead, she internalised a message that she wasn't important enough for anyone to notice her. Now craving comfort, Emily remembered that she was indeed self-centred. It seems that the external factors outside of Emily's control, present at the start of the crisis, had retreated into the shadows. Now she took sole responsibility for creating this interminable situation.

## SUICIDAL

When Emily called a doctor friend who was training in psychiatry, and told her that she felt suicidal, she didn't anticipate the consequences. Emily didn't actually *want* to die; there was no sense to her suicidal thoughts given her loving family and good prospects for the future. It was just that she didn't know how to make the nightmare stop and at that precise moment Emily felt desperate. But her desperation was to feel listened to, to be taken seriously and to feel better. This was no fantasy or story, but it escalated out of control in a similar way to when the police were called, when Emily was eight years old.

## OLD MANOR

It was a cold, bleak day in January 1995 and already dark, as Peter drove Emily to Salisbury. Earlier he had chauffeured her to an emergency assessment with the on-call psychiatrist at the Royal South Hants Hospital. From there, they had been instructed to stop home only briefly, to pack a few necessities as Emily needed admission at the Old Manor psychiatric hospital forty minutes away in Salisbury. Neither of them said a word during the journey. Emily was mesmerised by the windscreen wipers clearing the drizzle on the windscreen. She shivered not just from the cold, but from the knowledge that psychiatrists held power over her, and she had no choice. Resistance was futile. The psychiatrist told her how much better it was to be a 'voluntary' patient. "It's in your best interests," he had said.

Peter carried Emily's bag as they walked into the reception area at the Old Manor hospital. They were escorted to a small interview room where a white-coated junior doctor joined them. Peter was asked to leave; nobody explained anything to him and he drove home to the children feeling as afraid for their future as Emily felt for her own.

Peter's departure seemed like a short cut to Emily's four-year-old self, staring through the window at nursery school as her mother drove away. She tried to pay attention to the questions the young doctor was asking but she answered as an automaton, quietly and without inflexion to her speech. She became conscious of the spartan hospital furniture, its uniformity, and its lack of character. The drabness matched her feelings and then perhaps she could have been back in the school dormitory as much as at the nursery school window. She'd blown it again, this time by admitting to suicidal feelings. It was too late for regret. She could not avoid the consequences. She'd just been incarcerated as a mental patient and her life was in ruins.

## LOCALITY-SPECIFIC SYMPTOMS

It wasn't until the early 2000s that Emily reported her *locality-specific* reactions and fears, symptoms which are often labelled as PTSD. Her psychiatrists didn't pay much attention to what she was saying. One of the places where this consistently happened was as she passed the Old Manor hospital in Salisbury, usually on the way to visit her parents. She always tried to avoid driving past the site of the old Victorian hospital buildings because just catching sight of the hospital tower with its clock face, visible just above roof height, sent shivers down her spine. She felt her chest thumping rapidly and tightening the grip on the steering wheel, she had to keep her eyes fixed on the road ahead and determinedly stick to the thirty-mile-per-hour limit. Only as the building receded into the distance would she feel safe that the lingering menace could not touch her anymore.

While Emily learned to avoid being in the vicinity of the hospital where she had been a patient, she sensed a brush-off from her psychiatric team. Perhaps she was not the only one who favoured avoidance. Perhaps they would rather she didn't invade their territory. Perhaps when they told her it was a good thing that she'd lost memories as a result of ECT (electroconvulsive therapy), it had more sinister implications. The fact that the unknown remains unknown doesn't make it good or right.

In 2019, it was only a modicum of relief to discover that the old hospital had been razed to the ground. In its place, billboards advertised the new luxury flats. But to Emily, Old Manor is the home of ghosts. Even the new development is a reminder of its existence, imprisoned deep within Emily's psyche. Her body remembers, and it seems unlikely that it will ever forget. The rebuilding releases her from the possibility of ever setting foot on the premises again, but not from the necessity of facing up to the memories which remain.

## ECT

During the seven years from 1994 – 2001, Emily was given over one hundred separate ECT 'treatments', during which an electrical current, a 'shock' is passed through the brain via electrodes on either side of the head to intentionally induce a seizure. The first ECT Emily had was at the Old Manor hospital.

The consultant psychiatrist sought to allay her fears when he suggested ECT, shortly after her admission. He reassured her that she wouldn't feel a thing because she would be asleep under anaesthetic. Although no one could explain why it worked, Emily was told it would hasten her recovery and she would get better much more quickly than with medication alone. How could she say no to that?

To prevent violent muscle contractions during the seizure, a drug called suxamethonium is given to temporarily paralyse the patient during the procedure. Usually, it wears off within just three minutes. But on Emily's first ECT it did not wear off and she remained paralysed. She couldn't even breathe on her own and the anaesthetist had to hand-ventilate her lungs. He correctly suspected that she had a rare genetic enzyme deficiency which delayed the metabolism of this particular drug. He didn't know how long she would remain paralysed for. In extreme cases it could be for over twenty-four hours.

What Emily remembers is waking, to find herself surrounded by a group of very worried doctors and nurses. Subsequent blood tests confirmed that she did indeed have 'suxamethonium apnoea'.

After this near disaster, they continued the ECT using lower doses of the same drug, something I now find unbelievably irresponsible. Invariably Emily woke with a headache, totally disorientated, and it could take an hour or more before she regained her bearings. She suffered profound and permanent memory loss as a direct result of the ECT, which makes it impossible to know whether there was more to it than what she remembers of this one episode. Whatever happened, it traumatised her so badly that she continued to be affected decades later.

## MEDICATION CHANGES

The consultant psychiatrist made the first of numerous alterations to Emily's drug regimen. He started another older type of antidepressant called a 'tricyclic', as well as chlorpromazine, a very sedating drug used in the treatment of psychosis and therefore classed as an 'antipsychotic'. Emily tried to make notes and her scribbles provide valuable insight for that period of time.

## SIDE EFFECTS

It's clear that the many drugs she took caused many adverse effects (also known as side effects). Despite the sedating properties of chlorpromazine, she still couldn't sleep. She felt very restless with a horrible feeling in her limbs, as though they didn't want to keep still and she wrote how the room seemed to keep changing in size. She felt numb, as though everything was unreal. Her mouth was very dry, and though she welcomed drinks, it was embarrassing when the cup and saucer rattled, because she was unable to control the trembling of her shaky hands, and she kept spilling tea down her front. Other patients were kept waiting outside the bathroom when she had severe constipation and then the reverse happened, and her bloated tummy gave way to diarrhoea. She had no more energy than before she went into hospital; although she couldn't get to sleep, paradoxically she found it hard to get up in the morning and felt like a zombie all day.

The medical notes made no mention of oversedation, an obvious adverse effect of her cocktail of medication, and her slowness is reported as 'psychomotor retardation' another feature of depression, when it could also have been a side effect.

## DISCHARGED

After six weeks, Emily was discharged. She greeted the children after their day at school and asked them what they had done that day, as though nothing was unusual. Already an expert when it came to hiding her true feelings, Emily tried to behave as normally as possible. She wrote that there were times when she pottered around the house, getting the laundry done, tidying away the children's toys and felt almost back to normal. But she was very worried by the memory loss. She described work as a nightmare, and in capitals wrote, 'AND IT'S ALL MY FAULT'.

Despite Emily's reported suicidality, the psychiatrists were clearly not worried enough to restrict her prescriptions for the dangerous tricyclic antidepressants. When she complained that she didn't feel any better, she was told the antidepressants were still having 'some effect', which ensured her compliance. Emily was terrified of feeling worse and didn't dare omit doses of medication. She was in no danger of stockpiling the tablets.

Diary entries from that time reflect on her dilemma: if she disclosed how bad she was feeling, her ongoing suicidality and quasi plans to end it all, she would be readmitted to hospital and given more ECT. She hated hospital and the children also hated it when she was away from home. As time went on, ECT erased her memories of their tears, but she repeatedly wrote that she wanted the children to know she still loved them.

## DIAGNOSIS

The psychiatrists were convinced that Emily was suffering from a severe episode of major depression. Now she was well-established on antidepressants, she certainly ticked all the diagnostic criteria, although this wasn't the case *before* she started taking them.

Perhaps this is a moot point since there are no tests which can confirm or disprove a psychiatric diagnosis. Psychiatric diagnoses are made on the basis of a patient's directly reported symptoms, the doctor's observations of the patient's behaviour and their interpretations of the patient's answers to fairly standard questions. In depression, the diagnostic criteria include feelings of sadness, crying, obsessing over negative thoughts and loss of enjoyment – all considered abnormal if they have been present for 'most of the time' for more than an arbitrary two weeks. Other vague and non-specific symptoms include a *loss* or *gain* of appetite, *loss* or *gain* of weight, tiredness, low energy, sleeping *too little* or *too much* and sexual dysfunction. With the exception of dementias and a few other recognisable organic brain disorders, psychiatry continues to lack any physical confirmatory tests or investigations despite decades of research.

Yet since her first admission, Emily had been prescribed a cocktail of drugs, which could easily cause many of these symptoms. Furthermore, suddenly stopping antidepressants often causes withdrawal, which can be mistaken as a return of the original symptoms. But this was not common knowledge when Emily abruptly stopped Prozac after the first prescription.

## DEPARTMENT OF PSYCHIATRY

Doctors who require psychiatric admissions were routinely treated in a different area to where they worked, hence the reason Emily was initially admitted in Salisbury. But after the second admission, it was considered unlikely that Emily would recover sufficiently to return to work any time soon; her psychiatric care was transferred back to Southampton which made travel easier for the family.

On Emily's first admission to the DOP (Department of Psychiatry), at the Royal South Hants Hospital in Southampton, someone on the staff betrayed her confidentiality. The patients' dining room provided the perfect opportunity for some amusement at Emily's expense. Some patients took it in turns to sneak up behind her and whisper, "What's up, Doc?", before melting away in fits of laughter.

Losing her anonymity was bad enough, but life on the ward seemed unbearable when some of the nursing staff openly showed their disdain. Feeling shamed and worthless, Emily's symptoms spiralled. It seemed that her condition had become everyone's business: friends, family, and acquaintances all had a view.

## PARENTAL CONCERN

Emily's parents were also bewildered. George, her father, never understood emotional distress and he wanted answers. Having read in the newspaper that the same anti-malarial, Lariam, that the family had taken on their recent trip to the Philippines, could cause depression – unbeknown to her – he wrote to Emily's psychiatrist. He didn't receive a reply. It seems that none of her doctors even considered this a realistic cause of her original symptoms.

But Emily didn't see her father's concerns. Since they never talked at anything more than a superficial level, when he commented on how well she looked, Emily assumed he thought she was malingering. Trying hard to maintain a mask and put on a good front socially, the effort to conceal her depressive feelings became a double jeopardy. Emily hated all of it.

## STIGMA

When the psychiatrists told Emily that she was seriously ill as a result of 'endogenous' or biological depression, she felt validated. But the initial relief soon dissipated because it did not stop stigmatising attitudes towards her. The repeated reassurance that her severe major depression would get better with drugs and ECT ensured that she was fully compliant with treatment. In addition to this, she was mindful of the stipulations from the GMC (General Medical Council), that doctors who are unwell must follow the medical advice offered by those providing their care.

Yet the more treatment Emily received, the worse she felt. At the time, she didn't realise that all the diagnosis did was deflect attention away from the very real and significant, underlying causes of her problems.

In some respects, anti-stigma campaigns have made mental illness/ psychiatric diagnoses more acceptable. But as Emily found to her cost, while the focus remains centred on finding the right drugs to push the psychiatric condition into remission, a perception remains that people never fully recover. Friends and even some of her relatives seemed to have given up on Emily as soon as she was hospitalised for the first time. All she needed was a little bell and some rags to wear while she shouted, "Unclean, unclean." It was noticeable how quick people were to look the other way after the briefest, forced smile at church on Sundays.

* * *

*Do you think there may be different ways to improve your situation beyond your medical/psychiatric diagnosis? Perhaps there are other factors that could be taken into consideration. I would encourage you to nurture your curiosity.*

# CHAPTER 12

# Life as an inpatient

As I researched to write *Life After Darkness*, I plunged into Emily's diaries, consulted the tabletop family planners where Emily's admissions and appointments were recorded alongside all the children's activities. Some of the memories I retained from this period were vague and disjointed, others I can still recollect with terrifyingly vivid clarity.

PETER

The NHS is generous with regards to sick pay, but after six months it was apparent that Emily wasn't going to recover, so Peter had to find work. Emily held herself responsible, another cogent reminder of how hopeless the situation was.

Acts like peeling potatoes seemed to consume all Emily's energy, but she did her best to prepare the meal and cajole the children to do their homework before Peter arrived home after his long commute to work. The family always sat around the dining table to eat the evening meal together and then Emily tried to get her younger ones bathed, ready for bed and stories read before collapsing onto the sofa in the sitting room with Peter. Try as she might, she no longer felt close to anyone including her loving husband. There was little to distract Emily from her inner world, other than her feeble attempts to care for the children.

Thankfully Emily was not under the care of Dr Nas for long. She made the mistake of telling him how hard it was at home when Peter was laid up, having ruptured his Achilles tendon. Instead of being sympathetic to the situation, Dr Nas accused Peter of being selfish. Peter! The person who ran their household single-handed when Emily was in hospital. Peter, who organised for the children to be picked up and taken to all their activities every day after school. Peter, who had little time for his own self-care. Peter, who did everything while working full-time and commuting sixty miles by car to and from Guildford every day. He was a remarkable man, totally committed to the welfare of his family. Emily wasn't aware that he was also terrified that if he failed to provide for their needs, social services would take the children away.

Even though she was horrified and angry by what Dr Nas had said, Emily said nothing. Under normal circumstances, she would have spoken up and defended Peter to the hilt against such insults, but she had changed. She sat on the orange plastic chair looking at the brown carpet tiles, unassuming, uncomplaining, and compliant. She wished she'd never mentioned it and knew she must be careful what she said about home in the future. She left the appointment with another reason to feel guilty, not knowing how often Peter was near to despair, wondering how it was all going to end.

## FAITH IN PSYCHIATRY

News of Emily's misfortune had spread, and she even received unsolicited advice from neighbours who she hardly knew. But

Emily still had faith in the psychiatrists and believed that she was receiving the best care possible – she was completely dependent on her healthcare providers for information on the benefits and harms of drug treatment, and she was not offered alternatives. She did not know that the 'serotonin' theory of depression was purely hypothetical and that there was no concrete evidence to back it up. Indeed, most of the medical profession widely believed the myth that mental illnesses were 'brain conditions' needing treatment to correct a chemical imbalance. This was the theoretical foundation which led Emily's psychiatrists to prescribe one drug after another, when she failed to get better.

The effect was to *cause* a chemical imbalance as the drugs literally tinkered with the levels of multiple neurotransmitters including serotonin, dopamine, and noradrenalin in Emily's brain. Presumably her psychiatrists had not yet understood that brain and nerve cells adapt, altering the number of receptors on which these drugs and neurotransmitters act, in an attempt to maintain homeostasis.

For years on end, Emily was very lethargic, she had so little energy and when at home, hardly left the house. She consistently reported feelings of unreality and numbness. Her psychiatrists *always* put these symptoms down to depression. Yet these same symptoms, along with the tremor, restlessness, dizziness, constipation, dry mouth, and low libido, could easily have been attributed to the adverse effects of her prescribed medications. Her body was constantly awash with drugs which interfered with the way her brain and nervous system functioned. But Emily completely trusted her psychiatrists; she had no reason to know that the prevailing theories arose out of educated guesswork, and they had no scientific basis for the 'trial and error' approach they took to the many changes of her medication. Likewise, she never suspected that there was no real evidence behind the ECT they were so determined that she should have. Every time Emily was told about a modification to the treatment plan it was accompanied with optimism, always encouraging Emily that the new combination would provide the key to make her better. The justification for starting her on 'depot' antipsychotic injections like Depixol was to alleviate persistent suicidal thoughts. It was never successful, and in fact, Emily's self-harm became more frequent. In reality nothing made any headway and Emily gradually deteriorated. She clung to the psychiatrists' opinions, believing that she had a serious biological depression, hoping that there would be an improvement, while her inner narrative continuously bombarded her with thoughts that she wasn't fit to be alive.

The more entrenched the situation became the more hopeless she became. Emily regularly asked herself whether she was doing all she was asked, perplexed that having sought help from the right people, taken all the medical advice on offer, nothing got better. Her memory was shot to pieces and Emily assumed that she must be the problem.

## INSTITUTIONALISED

As Emily spent more and more time in hospital, to all intents and purposes she had become institutionalised in a very similar way to her childhood experience of boarding school. Whether sectioned (detained against her will) or not, she was effectively a prisoner on a locked ward. But unlike school, for most of the day there was nothing to do. Time was marked only by drinks, meals, and queuing up for medication. As Emily's sense of isolation increased so the construct of hopelessness and failure ran in parallel, and she had little reason to question her inner dialogue. Despite their best intentions, psychiatry simply reinforced all Emily's pre-existing negative and dysfunctional beliefs about herself.

When the diagnosis was revised to 'treatment-resistant depression', Emily was referred to Professor James West, the head of the mood disorders service in Southampton. He was kind and sympathetic to Emily's plight, as he added some fairly unusual drugs, hoping to enhance the antidepressant effect of those she was already taking. Already on the depot antipsychotics, Emily was started on Lithium as a mood stabiliser. Severe side effects including persistent lethargy continued and she gained a debilitating tremor, and also became hypothyroid. When the drug combinations didn't work, doses were increased, or another drug added or substituted. The possibility of stopping them altogether was never considered.

Despite losing memory through ECT, I can easily recollect conversations when Emily was coerced into giving her consent, including overt threats that if she failed to agree, she would be sectioned. Emily was first put on a section of the Mental Health Act that mandated treatment in 1996, although a special application had to be made to force her to have ECT against her will.

The perspective and clarity she had when she first sought help from her GP were gone. The original circumstances and the reawakening of childhood memories that caused her original crisis now seemed irrelevant. Sedated, muddled, and confused after regular ECT, Emily found it difficult to think coherently.

## BIOLOGICAL

Over and over again, Emily's psychiatrists reiterated their own theories about her very 'biological' illness, an 'endogenous depression' and Emily acquiesced to their views. Despite the side effects, she readily complied with the drugs, desperate to feel better, and absolutely terrified she might feel worse if she didn't. Her world had shrunk and felt unreal as she wore her chemical straitjacket without any insight that how she was feeling was directly related to the effects of her psychiatric drugs. Instead, she deferred to the experts and listened to the psychiatrists' explanation that she was experiencing 'derealisation' and 'depersonalisation' – further evidence of severe depression.

But as the years passed, Emily began to hear dissenting opinions, primarily from nurses on the ward. Some of them clearly didn't agree with her psychiatrists and were vocal of their scepticism. They accused Emily of *not wanting* to get better.

## THE WARD

There were five wards at the DOP (Department of Psychiatry). Most were set up in the same pattern, two corridors of separate dormitories, one male, one female, linked at one end by a large dayroom for both genders. A TV dominated one end of the room with chairs making a semicircle around it. Other plastic-covered easy chairs lined the walls, and there were a few rectangular coffee tables. The carpet was a dirty blue colour and many of the chairs were orange. The walls were a neutral colour, and could do with a fresh coat of paint; there were no pictures but the odd faded or torn poster conveyed various forgettable bits of information deemed useful for the patients to be aware of. Emily came to loathe the noise of endless game shows which emanated from daytime TV.

## ACTING UP

At least once a day, some kind of drama would break the monotony as frustrated patients started shouting or swearing at staff or one another. Often this would deteriorate into physical violence which brought the nursing staff rushing out of the office demanding them all to calm down. Usually this was ineffective and the patient or patients concerned would be rewarded with a chemical cosh; lorazepam was often the drug of choice.

Lisa, a lady in her fifties, was usually quiet and peaceable, so it seemed completely out of character when she suddenly upturned all the furniture. Later she admitted to Emily that she quite deliberately 'acted up' (as the nurses called it) because nobody had paid her any attention for days.

The only other place left for patients to go was to their beds in the six-bedded dormitories. Emily spent a lot of her day in her bedspace. She came to hate the brown flowery curtains which were the only form of privacy. Nursing staff knew she preferred to have a bed beside the window, where at least she could look out on the car park several storeys below, but it soon became a way that some of them could bully her. Jean, a fellow patient, remembers how as if on a whim, a nurse would come in and suddenly gather up all Emily's belongings from the window bed and dump them on a different bed, telling Emily she had to move. While she was victimised in this way, it further increased Emily's feelings of insecurity and her sense of worth plummeted.

Sometimes these same nurses would make up Emily's bed with only one thin blanket and she would be too cold to sleep. But when she asked for another one, she would be told there weren't any or there would be a substantial delay before her request was met. There was nowhere else to go and nowhere to hide. These micro-aggressions had the desired effect. Emily felt punished, her super-sensitised brain took it all on board. She didn't feel heard, and she certainly didn't feel understood, and the less compassionate the staff were towards her, the more convinced she became that she was a terrible failure, responsible for her disastrous life.

## CHURCH

When Emily was not in hospital, she still went to church. She was desperate for comfort from somewhere and asked for prayer on many occasions. At first, Emily was open about what was going on and shared her thoughts with the Christians she looked up to and trusted. But when prayer didn't improve the situation, the implication was that it was 'hidden sin' that prevented God from healing her. As memories from the past surfaced and her inner world was bombarded with everything that had gone wrong, Emily examined every motive; she begged God for forgiveness for every fault she could find. Leaders, elders, and many others prayed for her on multiple occasions, yet she didn't get better, which further evidenced that she was the problem, preventing God from intervening.

It seemed that wherever Emily turned, the message was always the same. It didn't matter how much she was suffering – at some deep level, she only had herself to blame. Even today, this element exists in our culture when we talk about people 'needing to take responsibility for themselves'. In this setting, Emily took her responsibility extremely seriously.

As time went on Emily came to believe she was unfit to exist. Thankfully for most of the time, this belief was tempered by her conviction that the children still needed their mother however fallible she was. But the more time she spent in hospital, away from home, the more hopeless it became. It is hard to describe the pain of such deep despair.

## KEEPING HOME

Peter had more than enough to cope with and even though he now had a full-time job, he and Emily were still experiencing financial pressure. During hospital admissions, the psychiatrists recognised that it was good for Emily to spend time at home with the children on a daily basis. It was a logistical nightmare for Peter to bring her home for the evening meal, driving through the rush hour traffic. He had to bring the children with him and then leave them in the car, while he collected Emily from the locked ward. Once home, he had to prepare the meal and afterwards, take Emily back to the hospital. Sometimes Emily resented Peter's kindness simply because it reinforced her own feelings of ineptitude.

In fact, as a couple, they were hardly communicating, each in their own way trying to protect the other and any conversation was usually restricted to practicalities. Living in a perpetual state of tension, it often spilled over into bickering and petty arguments. Thankfully Peter's work was sympathetic when it came to family emergencies such as one of the children falling sick, but he relied heavily on a network of a few faithful friends, as well as his mother and Emily's parents, who helped out. During term time, there was also a journey up to London every weekend to fetch Rachel and then take her back to White Lodge on Sunday evening. Is it any wonder that relationships were strained? Peter felt like an automaton.

Maybe to an outsider it might seem amazing that there were still regular occasions which the whole family enjoyed. Saturday evenings were always a bit of a tradition. Peter cooked homemade pizza which they ate together in the sitting room while they laughed their way through *Noel's House Party*. Harry, the youngest, liked to be on the floor with half his body tucked beneath the coffee table. For several years, they managed a summer holiday, driving to camp sites in France or Spain. During these breaks, the family were sufficiently distracted to forget about their ordeal for a brief couple of weeks at the beach, enjoying the Mediterranean weather.

It was unusual for long-term psychiatric patients in the DOP to stay with their partners. From the entries in Emily's medical notes, it is clear that the psychiatric team questioned Peter's motives because he continued to support Emily, his wife. Undoubtedly, Peter was truly remarkable, willing to sacrifice his own needs in his dedication to keep the family going, and Emily was extremely lucky to be married to someone who continued to love her despite it all. Maybe those short periods of respite were enough to prevent him from caving in.

## STAFF REPORTS

Pain of any nature varies in intensity and every human on the planet experiences the same phenomenon when it comes to emotion. In general, emotional pain is far more dependent on relationships with other people than the experience of physical pain but it is completely natural for our mood states to oscillate, even when it appears unpredictable to others. It was profoundly disempowering when staff placed more value on their individual judgements about what Emily was feeling than what she reported to them – the whole discipline of psychiatry relies solely on patients' self-reported symptoms. The psychiatrists rely on what a patient reports, and their own assessment on what they see is purely subjective because there is no real way of measuring emotions or feelings. But what gets recorded in the medical or nursing record is heavily dependent on the member of staff concerned. Worse still, Emily discovered that when she was not believed, she was simultaneously being labelled as manipulative.

Emily: "I'm not feeling so good right now."

Nurse: "But the notes say that the weekend went really well. You watched a film with the children."

Emily: "Yes, I did. But I'm feeling really low again."

Nurse: "But you said you had a good weekend."

This kind of circular argument was not uncommon, and it left Emily feeling guilty because *she wondered if her moments of respite must signify that staff were right and actually, she was a fraud.* While Emily thought some of the nurses were mean, she couldn't shake off what they said.

It was really hard for her to be caught up in such hostile internal dialogue. She was so full of self-doubt, and yet desperate to be vindicated. She didn't know who she could trust, and it often felt as though the detail of her life was under a microscope. Sleep was the only respite from constant torment, but the diurnal rhythm was eliminated by medication. Despite sleeping tablets, Emily was often awake in the middle of the night, groggy and worn out during the day.

This continued for years despite multiple alterations to the drug regime. The only thing that changed was the nature of the unpleasant side effects she was forced to endure. On every hospital admission, Emily was given more ECT. After ten – twelve treatments, usually it was recorded that her mood had improved but since it caused severe memory loss, how could anyone be sure? Without question, any improvement was never sustained, and the cycle continued. By 2001, Emily was put on 'maintenance' ECT.

After five or six years, the initial diagnosis of major depression was revised to include psychotic features, based on the fact that she started to hear discordant music. It was a strange phenomenon, like a child playing a mouth organ badly; thankfully it was intermittent, unlike the continuous negative self-beliefs that she was bad, a failure and to blame, deemed to be part of a nihilistic delusional state and further evidence of psychosis.

## SUICIDALITY ON ANTIDEPRESSANTS

Emily had never harboured any suicidal thoughts or contemplated harming herself before she started on antidepressants. While it is impossible to prove what role the drugs played in her deterioration, it is highly probable that the medicalisation of her distress and the false promises that antidepressants and ECT would make her better, fuelled Emily's downward spiral.

* * *

*Please do not lose heart, even though there is more to come before Emily had a breakthrough. If you or your loved one feel as though your own situation is hopeless with no light on the horizon,* remember that you are not alone and that even out of the ashes, a phoenix may arise!

Some people do feel better while taking antidepressants, often attributed to the numbing effect which may take the edge off particularly intense depressive feelings. Do you feel better taking psychiatric drugs? Recently, publicity has been given to the meta-analysis from Professor Joanna Moncrieff et al, which demonstrated that there is no evidence of long-term effectiveness for antidepressants. WARNING: psychiatric drugs should NOT be stopped suddenly. It may lead to severe and/or persistent withdrawal symptoms. If you want to stop your medication, please seek help from your doctor.

# CHAPTER 13

# Psychotherapy

As a patient, Emily was quiet and undemonstrative and left to her own devices for days on end, her negative and distressing thoughts went unfettered. As the rumination continued, they only grew in strength and intensity. It seems obvious now, that no amount of medication or ECT would solve Emily's internal conflicts and emotional problems, compounded as they were by her experiences as a psychiatric inpatient.

## ROOT CAUSES

Even though Emily was referred for psychotherapy right from the start of her initial crisis in the winter of 1994, it seems that her psychiatrists didn't hold any hope that it would provide answers. Even the psychotherapists failed to give any credence to the possibility that her emotional crisis, manifesting in the symptoms diagnosed as depression, could be directly related to the psychological injury and the emotional neglect she experienced at boarding school.

When Emily talked about her painful memories during

therapy sessions, she would be asked "and how does that make you feel?"

But Emily was unable to answer coherently because the drugs given to treat her depression, had numbed her emotions. Antidepressants prevented her from accessing feelings related to the past and Emily felt as if she had been wrapped in cling film and it made it impossible to articulate exactly how she felt about anything.

## SERENA

Even so, Emily valued the sessions because it was the only chance she had to talk about what was happening to her. After a couple of years, a more experienced therapist, Serena, took over Emily's psychotherapy.

In retrospect, it hardly seems surprising that the more Emily talked about her painful childhood, the worse she felt. Rationally, Emily had always maintained that however much she hated her schooling, her parents had still done their best for her. She felt no justification to hold them to account even though they were responsible for her. Occasionally she had the odd flash of anger when she blamed them for not listening to her, but it was transient, like a plume of fire hissing out from an active volcano. Deep inside, the tension bubbled beneath the surface, yet with her emotions so dumbed down by antidepressants, the volcano never erupted and there was no relief from the pressure.

I am not sure when Emily became aware that Serena was trying to uncover something deeper, more than she had already talked about. It seems that the psychiatrists and therapists had come to the joint conclusion that nothing she had disclosed so far, was serious enough to account for the treatment failure. As a result of this erroneous interpretation, they pushed Emily further, hoping to uncover repressed sexual abuse, which she never suffered.

Emily was tempted to get it over with by making something up, just to get them off her back, but she knew she must stay totally honest. However, it was disconcerting, and Emily found herself wondering if perhaps there was some dark secret she wasn't aware of, buried in her psyche. She dug deep and offered up each and every possible bad memory from her childhood. Maybe it was this quest for non-existent repressed memories, that blindsided Emily's therapists so much that they failed to give sufficient weight to the possibility of serious psychological injury arising from her experiences of boarding school.

Sadly, many female patients who disclose childhood sexual abuse earn themselves a label of personality disorder which further stigmatises these vulnerable women. Emily met some lovely women on the ward who after years of discriminatory 'treatment', delivered by those who were paid to help them, were then written off as incurable and discharged from psychiatric services.

## CONSTANCY

When Serena finally stopped delving into her past, Emily was still encouraged to share what was on her mind. But their interactions reminded her of the rare conversations she had had as an adolescent with adults around her; they always gave such logical answers. Emily desperately wanted compassion, she needed an empathic response to what she shared. Yet the two therapists were the most consistent people assigned to her throughout the whole seven-year period. There had been many different consultant psychiatrists, junior doctors and CPNs (community psychiatric nurses) assigned to Emily's case; and even when she was lucky enough to have sympathetic nurses on the ward, they were constantly chopping and changing.

On the ward, patients were allocated a maximum of thirty minutes once a week to talk with their key nurse and all too often they were too busy to fulfil this task. It must have been demoralising for these trained nurses, when the sole purpose of the ward seemed to be as a detention centre, where their main function was to dispense medication four or five times a day to the queue of waiting patients. The ward was very far removed from being a therapeutic environment.

After each therapy session, Emily, the expert at rumination, would carry on cogitating over what had been discussed. Although she often expressed her belief that she was to blame and had ruined everything, she cannot remember anyone trying to persuade her otherwise. Whether her therapists or psychiatrists cogently and persistently contradicted her false narrative or not, there were enough people who reinforced her self-denigration. Her continued deterioration, however gradual, provided Emily with ample proof that she was a failure as a wife, a mother, a doctor, a daughter, a sister and as a Christian. But the psychiatrists saw Emily's logical conclusion as evidence of a nihilistic delusion and attributed it to psychotic depression.

## PARALLELS

In 2017, Barb pointed out how easy it was to see the parallels between Emily's admissions to hospital and her time at boarding school. It was startling and now seems so obvious. But when I researched Emily's medical record, I could find nothing which linked Emily's 'current' situation to her past experiences as a boarding school survivor.

When hospitalised, Emily's freedom was curtailed. Even as a 'voluntary' patient, she resided on a locked ward, never free to come and go as she pleased. She was bullied by patients and staff, and when she tried to express what she was feeling, she didn't feel listened to. The majority of the time Emily slept in a dormitory and the food was institutional. Some of the nurses' behaviour could be likened to the tyrannical matrons, while the psychiatrists seemed more akin to the largely benign teachers of her school days. Emily was usually discharged from hospital in time to coincide with the school holidays when her children were at home. Then once term started again, another admission soon followed.

Barb's hypothesis made perfect sense, especially because the admissions had such a well-established temporal pattern. The psychiatrists rationalised that this pattern was because Emily felt drained after the exertion of looking after the children during the school holidays. I wonder why alternatives were not considered and that the connections to Emily's past childhood trauma were not made at that time.

## AIR TRAVEL

I have also wondered why the psychotherapists failed to be impressed when Emily described what had become a Pavlov-type response to the sound of the engines revving for take-off on plane journeys. She told them how she still cried even when they were going away for a family holiday. The tears were triggered as soon as the hum of the plane engines became the screech just before the plane starts its thunderous journey down the runway. Even decades after the distraught journeys back to boarding school, her attempts to assert mind over matter had failed. As an adult, Emily would choose a window seat to concentrate on watching the ground spin away from under her, while she fought hard to hold back tears which appeared as automatically as the wheels being drawn back into the body of the plane.

## UNDESERVING

Of course, therapists and psychiatrists hear terrible stories of horrendous abuse that so many of the world's children have endured through no fault of their own. Emily made her own comparisons about what had happened to her as a child. She thought she had no right to feel the way she did, which increased her inner conviction that she was both weak and selfish. Perhaps attributional or confirmation bias was never considered when the psychiatrists repeatedly diagnosed major depression, rather than return to the beginning and look at it from a fresh perspective. Perhaps it was too difficult to back down from such a theory, after so many different treatments had been instigated.

I wonder why the severity of Emily's traumatic experiences and circumstances while she was growing up was not recognised. Maybe, like Emily, they completely forgot the reason why she sought help in the first place. Presumably they paid scant attention to the clues Emily left along the way. Perhaps the professionals charged with her care were just ignorant about the effects of emotional neglect or trauma on a person's life. Maybe they never thought to give it their attention or to research what was known to be the effects of boarding school on children. 'Boarding School Syndrome' was already in the public arena if they had cared to look.

* * *

*Some people are tempted to belittle the suffering of boarding school children because many come from privileged homes. But whatever your background, all children should be protected from abuse and neglect. Unrecognised, childhood adversity may wreak havoc in later life, leading to serious health problems and ruining the lives of other family members. What are the root causes of your problems? Can you think of any particular keys which might help unlock your current struggles?*

# CHAPTER 14

# Alert: self-harm

Self-harm may be a catch-all term when someone tries to procure an injury, ingest a harmful object or substance, or even intentionally withhold what is needed to be healthy. Yet it's easy to forget that the vast majority of adults knowingly hurt themselves from time to time, even if not for the same reasons. In the Western world they might smoke, drink, eat too much, drive too fast, not go to bed when tired, gamble, or spend too much money...

Some people are clear that they use self-harm as a coping mechanism, and they find it annoying when people encourage them to stop.

Self-harm may arise out of anger following an argument, or despair following the break-up of a relationship. It may be a trivial act but with the conviction that it may lead to death, or self-harm may have serious, unforeseen consequences. It may arise with genuine suicidal intent and then be regretted within a short space of time.

In the context of Emily's life as a psychiatric patient, the underlying reasons behind her self-harm event were not just complex, but also in a state of flux.

## CONTAGION

When Emily was at school, self-harm as we know it today, wasn't an entity. A few girls dieted excessively; others made themselves vomit but even that was relatively rare. Then as time went on, suicide became less taboo and was occasionally reported in the newspaper or on the news.

It has taken a while to establish that there is a direct relationship between the media reporting of a celebrity suicide and events such as fatal car crashes involving no one else. Likewise, the rate of overt suicides substantially increases in the days and weeks following… This phenomenon persists and has catastrophic consequences. Nowadays, social media has accelerated the plethora of copycat behaviours. This changes both the risk, as well as the demographic of those who self-harm.

In the setting of a psychiatric unit, where patients regularly engage in acts of self-harm, it becomes an atmosphere ripe for similar propagation of these events. But that is not the whole story.

## AKATHISIA

Nobody denies the reality of the suffering of those who are in deep depression. Yet, being harmed by the treatment that is supposed to help should never be part of the equation. While it is widely recognised that some psychiatric medications including antidepressants may cause increased thoughts of suicide and self-harm in children and young people, what is less well-known is that, although rare, they can also induce homicidal ideation. Likewise, but again uncommon, suicidal and/or homicidal thoughts and behaviours can also be linked to psychiatric drugs in adults. This can be mediated through a serious but rare side effect called akathisia. These effects have been seen in healthy volunteers without any prior history of mental health problems, but this information has been deliberately suppressed.

Some psychiatrists are worried because they think that antidepressants are useful drugs to treat depression and they do not want people to be deterred from taking them. But this logic cannot be maintained when there is very little evidence that antidepressants work. Yet publicity is weighted towards those people who report feeling better while taking these drugs, and undermines the stark reality that there is a risk for others of serious harm, and avoidable deaths may result.

This is an important principle for Emily's experience. She was never suicidal and never had any thoughts of self-harm prior to taking antidepressants.

## CURRENCY

Within the healthcare setting, self-harm, like violence, is a currency that staff understand. It always leads to a response. Psychiatrists often use rating scales to assess the severity of depression, likewise they assess their patients' level of distress by asking about the presence and seriousness of threats of self-harm or suicide. Even though it is notoriously difficult to predict which patients who self-harm or attempt suicide will eventually complete suicide at a later date, it has never stopped the psychiatric community from drawing up checklists and trying to devise ways of stratifying risk. Is it any wonder that patients who act on their suicidal thoughts soon learn that this will send a message to their healthcare team that they aren't doing so well?

However, those who self-harm too frequently, according to some arbitrary and subjective measure, will be suspected of having a 'borderline' or 'emotionally unstable' personality disorder. Once given that label, any subsequent self-harm behaviour is likely to be redefined as manipulative. This is a travesty when so many patients given a personality disorder diagnosis, have been sexually abused or neglected as children. They were damaged through no fault of their own and when psychiatric services admit they have little to offer, and deem them to be untreatable, is it any wonder that they feel rejected? It may then exacerbate any pre-existing difficulties they have in forming trusting relationships. Even though the risk of accidental death is high in such cases, little attention is paid either to the possibility that self-harm is an indication of unmet need or to the potential for recovery. It is a terrible indictment on the medical profession that people can be written off as hopeless cases, for such nebulous reasons.

## EMILY LISTENS

Emily heard this debate being played out amongst her own healthcare team. In some ways she was lucky that her psychiatrists were persistent in believing she suffered from treatment-resistant depression, because they did not give up on her. Yet some nurses who did not share their opinions, were both judgmental and punitive towards Emily.

She was constantly on the alert, vigilant as she sat in the dayroom for weeks on end. She had plenty of time to observe her fellow patients, overhear discussions on how to self-harm and witness the results of self-inflicted injury. Emily hated the pejorative views of the staff towards those who self-harmed, often dismissing them as 'attention-seeking'. There were far easier ways to draw attention to oneself. Why not dress up in a clown outfit? It betrayed such ignorance of the complicated factors that lead people to overcome their innate resistance to pain and injury. Emily's own requests for help were often ignored, and she lost faith in the staff when she was met with disinterest or a curt, "Not now, I'm busy."

## VARIOUS

Emily secretly hurt herself for the first time as early as 1995 while at home, and she didn't tell anyone about it. Nothing was helping, no one understood, and she didn't feel listened to.

During one admission, Emily spent months restricting what she ate. Effectively, she was on hunger strike. When I first viewed the medical record to write *Life After Darkness*, I was shocked to read the psychiatrists' hypotheses over why she wasn't eating. They would have saved themselves no end of trouble if they had discussed it with her straight off. Weeks later, when they finally asked, she answered honestly that she was trying to starve herself to death. Emily was sectioned which gave a legal basis to force her to have ECT against her will and she was made to take olanzapine. It was impossible to resist food under the influence of olanzapine – one of its side effects leads to a voracious appetite. In a short space of time, Emily went from being severely undernourished to obese.

Once home after this admission, Emily began to scald herself, often in the middle of the night. The severe pain of the burn served as punishment as well as useful distraction from persistent mental torment. Next, she experimented with cutting which she had seen so many other patients do. It was so easy. The first time she tried, it barely took five minutes to cut her arms multiple times; something she never did again and something she was to regret for the rest of her life. Now she was visibly marked, ironically the literal meaning of stigma; the scars made her into 'one of those people who self-harm'.

## INTENTION

Even though suicide seemed the only way out of her predicaments, Emily didn't want to die; she never wanted to abandon her family. She always wanted to see her children grow up and be part of their lives. Her real desire was for the nightmare to end and for life to return to normal. But as time went on, the situation escalated, and she truly believed that her husband and children would be better off without her. It is hard to describe the torment and anguish that didn't leave her except during sleep. During the sixth year, Emily was so utterly desolate, that she was rarely free from thoughts of self-harm and suicide. Although the intensity fluctuated, it was hard to resist the impulses to 'end it all'. (With easy access to firearms, it is easy to see why suicide is the highest cause of death by shooting in the USA.)

When Emily's section was renewed, she was permanently hospitalised. Opportunistically she managed to escape from the locked ward and took a potentially lethal cocktail of pills, procured at low cost from a local pharmacy. She sat in a café afterwards waiting for it to take effect; during the time lag, she felt guilty – this kind of ambivalence has saved many a patient after an overdose. Eventually she responded to one of the many frantic calls from Peter. It was her first A&E attendance resulting from self-harm.

When Emily self-harmed, she was not in a normal, rational state of mind. She didn't consciously use self-harm as a coping mechanism, although she saw that it was some kind of response to her internal world of protracted turmoil and torment. She had lost touch with reality in a way that remains incomprehensible to me now. While she didn't want the children to think she had caused her own death i.e. had left them voluntarily, she became sufficiently deluded that she thought if she died because of complications, it would not count as 'suicide'. This crazy idea became a fixed obsession, and thoughts of self-harm went round and round until she acted on them. Being detained on a section did nothing to terminate her profoundly mixed-up thinking, it just made carrying out each inherently risky act of self-harm more difficult.

## A&E PATIENT

Emily hated being taken to A&E and never took herself there voluntarily; she had valid reasons to be fearful about visiting the place where she used to work. Every occasion was a nightmare and filled her with shame. Like on the psychiatric ward where she was detained, she was often humiliated and subjected to further abuse from doctors and nurses who lacked insight and compassion to do otherwise. Not infrequently, she ended up being taken to the operating theatre to repair the damage she had inflicted on herself. The staff who believed punishment would deter further acts of self-harm failed to understand how it achieved the opposite of what they intended. It just ground Emily's self-esteem ever lower, with the result that she punished herself even more purposefully.

During one of the A&E visits, the surgical registrar was called again. The gaping wound was too deep and too complex for the doctors in A&E. He took a look. "Not for theatre this time."

He pushed the trolley she was lying on into the treatment room and shut the door. They were alone together. He was tall in his surgical scrubs, a white face, his hair hidden in a surgical cap. His name Emily cannot remember, his words she cannot forget.

"You weren't satisfied with my handiwork last time, is that it?"

He unwrapped his surgical instruments and pulled the needles from their sheaths. There was no local anaesthetic and Emily knew that he wanted her to suffer. He made no attempt to be gentle and yet he was meticulous, neat even, as he stitched up Emily's self-inflicted wound layer by layer, bleeding and sore. He had no intention of sparing her from pain when he himself had to suffer the indignity of having to deal with such a pathetic creature who was wasting his precious time, keeping him from his real job of helping the deserving patients, those who had real illnesses in need of his surgical skills.

How could Emily object? She couldn't cry out, yell, or scream when she agreed with him; she was responsible. It was all her fault. She merely whimpered as she endured and even though she admitted this was what she really deserved, the real payback would come later. Then she would berate herself ferociously, riling against herself for her stupidity, incompetence, and pure selfishness, which brought her back to A&E for yet another dose of humiliation. Why couldn't she do it properly? For sure, the near miss when she had gone into shock while she was bleeding internally, curtailed it for a while. She had felt her life draining into oblivion before she was resuscitated; it had been a dreadful experience.

## QUESTIONS

I have to ask myself how did it come to this? Emily, who had been in a good job, with a good marriage and four lovely children... How was it that educated, trained healthcare staff could possibly conclude that Emily wanted to be incarcerated on a locked ward in a psychiatric hospital? What could she possibly gain? What made them so blind to her distress, so indiscriminate in their condemnation that they simply could not see that "pull yourself together" or "just stop this ridiculous behaviour" was impossible. Emily knew she was ruining her life. She oscillated between thinking that her family was fine without her and the guilt of being a bad mother. Perhaps it was a blessing that she was unable to see just how badly it affected them. Either way, she was stuck in a dangerous and vicious cycle driven by an unknowable, irrational desire to injure herself so badly, that she would die. The longer it carried on, the worse it became, and she could see no way out.

But now she believed that if she succeeded and died, God would surely forgive her. The back and forth, the see-saw, the tension, as unbidden a reminder popped to the fore – *the children*, she simply couldn't forget about the children. *Every child needs their mother. Surely a bad mother was better than a dead one. Peter*, she rationalised, *can find a new wife.* She could be traded in for a better model, one that was neither sad, nor bad like she was. But a mother was irreplaceable. It was the children who kept Emily going.

Once she returned back to the ward at the DOP, staff wouldn't talk to Emily about it. Nobody asked how she was feeling. They weren't sympathetic and they didn't ask her what was driving her self-harm. It was the elephant in the room, never mentioned, never asked about. Perhaps they thought talking about it would encourage her to self-harm more. Yet some staff made no attempt to conceal their contempt, and the worse she was treated, the more determined Emily became to succeed with her suicide attempts. These staff didn't see Emily. They didn't know who she really was.

Staff didn't know where she got the blades from, but it didn't stop them accusing her of giving them to other patients. Emily thought they were such fools; apart from the fact that she would never enable or encourage other patients to harm themselves, she wasn't going to give away her precious blades. It had taken great ingenuity to obtain them in the first place.

Since then, I've heard lots about the reasons *why* people self-harm – you can read about it in a leaflet, alongside the 'solutions'...

But why did Emily self-harm to the extent that she was literally crazy?

## ANSWERS

The psychiatrists saw an illness, they didn't see her, the real person. They didn't see Emily in the context of her life, her family or what she had been through in the past –none of that was part of the picture. But what really drove her crazy was being repeatedly told the drugs and ECT would make her better, when all it did was give her horrible side effects.

Maybe self-harm was a distraction from mental torment.

Maybe self-harm was an outward sign of inner torment.

Maybe she wanted to draw attention to her inner torment.

Maybe she felt no one was listening.

Maybe it was purely punishment.

Maybe Emily wanted to die and furthermore, her brain was under the influence of a concoction of drugs and chemicals which altered the way she thought and felt about life. She was taking drugs which are known to cause self-harm and suicidal thoughts in some healthy volunteers. Who knows what part any of these reasons played in Emily's life at that time when she was desperate and overwhelmed.

## BENEFICIAL ACTION

The only thing Emily ever found helpful was being listened to without judgement. Once a kind nurse ran Emily a bubble bath and made her a mug of cocoa. But as with any painkiller, even 'being heard' wears off and it wasn't always there when it was needed, which actually means time and time again.

I wonder what would have happened if Emily had felt respected, instead of being infantilised, and treated like a naughty child. How did anyone really think it would help when she was repeatedly accused of hurting herself in order to stay in hospital? There was little respite from the contemptuous eye-rolling, head-shaking and disparaging remarks just loud enough so Emily would hear. There was no escape from the facile comments made by those paid to care for her twenty-four hours a day. The punishments continued while they refused to honour even minor requests; she was treated as though she was someone who had deliberately set out to misuse their services. It's incredible to believe that they thought she was a rational person at that time, in full control of her thoughts and feelings. Why would they believe she wanted to reside in the DOP rather than at home with her family? Did their attitudes help extinguish her agony and internal torment? Surely there were alternative ways to encourage her adult, independent self to come out of hiding.

## CONSEQUENCES

What she could never have predicted was that these acts of self-harm would have far-reaching consequences not just in the short term; it would continue to dog her for very many years to come, even following recovery.

When Emily returned to work in A&E in 2002, a nurse told her she should have known better. Not long afterwards she overheard a colleague say, "People who overdose deserve to be rodded." He meant the old-fashioned idea of having the stomach pumped. Even today derogatory comments about patients who self-harm still surface in healthcare settings.

On one occasion while giving a talk about my experiences, one of the participants asked a question. "But were you *really* suicidal? Surely you would have successfully killed yourself if you were!"

At the time, I felt offended considering all that I had shared, but it was a fair question. In retrospect I don't know how determined Emily was to act on her suicidal thoughts on *each and every* occasion she was sectioned. What I do know is that Emily *always* wanted help. She wanted to be rescued from her impossible situation. She wanted out. After several years of psychiatric treatment, she felt betrayed by empty promises. It fuelled her hopelessness, picking up the desperation the psychiatrists clearly felt as they scraped the bottom of the barrel, while they toyed with combinations of drugs, or further ECT, all with assurances that it would restore her to health, while everyone wondered how it would end.

I found it particularly disconcerting in a professional context to hear a consultant psychiatrist opine, "If a patient really wanted to kill themselves, there would be nothing we could do to stop them, hospitalised or not."

It led me to consider the question of whether it is ethical for a psychiatrist to hold such views and yet use their formidable powers to recommend the detention of suicidal patients under the Mental Health Act.

\* \* \*

*There may be potential for minor acts of self-harm to escalate into something very dangerous with a high risk of accidental death. But it is very important not to confront or remove underlying coping mechanisms until the person at the centre of concern feels ready and has adequate alternative support. It goes without saying that this should be completely voluntary. Are you someone who self-harms? Are you in a place to consider exploring what is happening in more detail? If not, it might be better to wait some more and perhaps find someone you can trust to give you support.*

# CHAPTER 15

# More on psychiatry

However compassionate the individual players are, the psychiatric profession is full of paternalism. Emily looked up to her psychiatrists. They always believed they were doing the right thing for their patients and gave their very best care, within the confines of the biomedical model of psychiatry to which they were dedicated. When they sectioned Emily, they did so 'in her best interests'. Nonetheless the revolving door admissions, especially during the times when Emily was detained on a section, have furnished her with some exquisitely painful memories. Some of these ghastly episodes feel as though they were burnt into her brain and etched onto her very being.

## AWAKE ECT

One of these events occurred during the time when Emily was forced to have ECT against her will. The ECT suite had rooms which were big enough to have a typical hospital stretcher plus a table on which sat the ECT box which delivered the electric shock. Although there was a suction unit, alongside an oxygen supply, there were no continuous monitors like there are in operating theatres or A&E resuscitation rooms. The nurse took periodic blood pressure and heart-rate readings. The anaesthetist was in charge of giving the drugs and kept an eye on oxygen saturations.

As usual, Emily was brought into the room by the nurse and asked to lie down on the stretcher. The anaesthetist was relaxed and chatted to the nurse as they took Emily's hand to insert the intravenous cannula into a vein, to give the drugs that would put her to sleep. Emily knew the drill. The tight-fitting oxygen mask was placed over her mouth and nose, and she was asked to take deep breaths while the anaesthetist injected the drugs. The rubbery smell of the mask wouldn't last long, and she would feel the pain going up her arm caused by propofol, (the drug injected to put her to sleep), as it goes through the veins and then she would drift into oblivion. But nothing happened and then the awful realisation dawned that she was still awake, but unable to move and that the anaesthetist hadn't noticed. Emily had obviously been given the drug which caused paralysis to stop the awful jerking of a seizure, but not the drug to send her to sleep – she was fully conscious. Paralysed, panic-stricken and petrified, Emily had no way of getting anyone's attention. The junior doctor connected the electrodes to the sides of her head, about to give her the electric shock. Then… Emily remembered nothing.

When she came round, Emily was beside herself. The nurse examined her red, swollen hand. Clearly the cannula had come out of the vein. Professor West, her consultant psychiatrist, believed her. He told her he knew Emily was telling the truth because she couldn't remember the actual moment of the electric shock. The seizure it provoked would have wiped her memory of it.

Emily didn't make a formal complaint, but Professor West arranged for the NHS to pay for private sessions of EMDR

(Eye Movement Desensitisation and Reprocessing) which was supposed to help her recover from the trauma. She never received any explanation for what had happened nor any apology from the anaesthetist. She never got over the trauma either.

## COMPLAINT

Emily only ever attempted a formal complaint once despite the regular abuses she suffered at the hands of the medical or nursing staff. After the managers investigated her allegations, they sent her a written reply. Emily opened the envelope and it felt like her stomach had been punched as she read a counter-accusation that she had shouted at the staff. It was completely false and despite the support of an advocate, Emily felt even more vulnerable. She totally lost trust in the system. Without confidence or energy to continue the fight, she took it no further.

When I went through Emily's medical records to write *Life After Darkness*, I found her letter of complaint and the manager's response filed in her notes for all to see. Hospital policy dictated that all complaints should be kept separate from the medical record. They had failed her again. Emily never stood a chance…

## PULL YOURSELF TOGETHER

It was about four years after the original crisis, when Emily returned home after a hospital admission and gave herself a stiff talking to. "Enough is enough, everyone is right, you've brought this on yourself. Pull yourself together. No more nonsense. Get back to work."

Decision made, Emily called on her considerable willpower, guts, and determination as she had done so successfully in the past. At her outpatient appointment, Emily told Professor West of her plans. Not unnaturally, he was doubtful and questioned the wisdom of it all but couldn't stop her from trying.

It was disappointing to discover that both of the A&E consultants Emily had worked for previously, had left. But Emily wasn't one to fall at the first hurdle. She made an appointment to meet the new head of department at Southampton General A&E. This consultant told Emily that she would need to spend some time as a clinical observer as the first step in her return to work. He sent her to HR (Human Resources) to get an honorary contract put in place, but HR said she would need Occupational Health clearance. They sent Emily to Occupational Health, where she was told she must first see one of their doctors to ensure she was fit to return to work. From that moment on, Emily knew it was futile because they would request a report from her psychiatrist.

Defeated, Emily went home, her world shattered. There was no way out. She was no doctor and never would be again. This was no ordinary downward spiral; Emily was riding the drill piece as it descended to the depths of hell and a permanent life as a psychiatric patient.

## SOCIAL SERVICES

There had been several stories in the media about the way heavy-handed social services had removed children from their homes without warning. It had terrified Peter and motivated him to make sure that family life continued as normally as possible while the children, one by one, entered the turmoil of adolescence. But Peter was also trying to survive himself, largely on his own, devoid of emotional support. Emily didn't realise how scared he was that any show of weakness on his part might lead to the children being taken into care. Neither did she see how excluded he felt when her psychiatrists left him out of any discussions over her treatment. She couldn't feel his anguish, but she saw his frustration and fatigue. The psychiatric team rarely exchanged words with him at all, but there was one occasion when Professor West invited the whole family to his office. Peter, Emily, and the children sat round his large conference table – hardly conducive to the 'chat' he wanted to have with them. The children didn't say a word. Most of the time, Emily was treated as a separate entity, far removed from the rest of her family.

## CHILDREN

When Natalie, their second daughter, also auditioned and was offered a place at the Royal Ballet School, finances became even tighter. Although the places were government grant assisted, they still had to give a means-tested contribution and other hidden costs were plentiful. Peter had a good job, yet their financial situation was dire, and he had to remortgage the house.

Looking back, it seems bizarre how little insight Emily had into the real situation at home. For years, she grossly underestimated the impact her condition had on the family. The mentally ill are stigmatised by society and so are their families as well. The children couldn't talk about what was happening to their mum either at school or with their friends. They were the secondary victims in the tragedy where their mother played the central character. Emily valued Peter's dedication to the family in caring for the children, but her low sense of self-worth tricked her into believing that she was just an additional burden for them all to carry.

## CHURCH COMMUNITY

At heart, the church community was both loving and supportive towards Emily's family, but they adhered to fundamentalist doctrines favoured by Protestant evangelicals which were at best, unhelpful. The dogma described how all people are sinners undeserving of God's love, but by believing that Jesus Christ died to pay the price for their sins, they would be forgiven. On Sundays, a preacher would expound the scriptures, encouraging strict adherence to biblical teachings and the congregation were frequently reminded of how they owed God unwavering gratitude and worship. Although some of the Christian beliefs had never sat well with Emily, by this stage in her life, she had been well and truly indoctrinated. Emily fully accepted the premise that she was born bad and without Christ she was nothing; there were many warnings against straying from biblical truths. In their church another popular teaching was that once 'saved', Christians were supposed to be the happiest people in the world. Clearly Emily wasn't anywhere near hitting the mark.

Church leaders and even the Christian doctors from Emily's GP practice, encouraged her to have faith in God's healing power. Yet when she presented herself for prayer, she found herself subjected to further scrutiny, unsolicited advice, and opinion. Commonly she was asked, "And how is your relationship with God?"

A significant number of Christians didn't believe in the concept of mental illness; they interpreted feelings of depression as a sign of spiritual sickness or like Emily's medical colleagues, a sign of character weakness. Many Christians suspected that a person who was depressed harboured unforgiveness or hidden sin and some even believed it was a sign of demonic oppression. She was asked about previous activities which might have given the devil access to her life.

The underlying judgement that rang in Emily's ears when she failed to get better was – 'God is perfect, therefore the fault must lie with you'. She craved comfort but the onus was always back on her.

By 2000, she no longer wanted anyone to pray for her, believing she was a hopeless case and a useless Christian, only fit for the scrap-heap. While she continued to believe in God, she also believed that if she died at her own hand, she would be forgiven. It gave her permission for suicide.

## TREATMENT OPTION

Professor West continued to make changes to her medication, which included a rarely used MAOI (monoamine oxidase inhibitor), for which she had to eliminate cheese and other foods from her diet, to avoid a dangerous reaction. He also added drugs which are not normally used in psychiatry, which it was hoped might enhance her existing medication. Sometimes Emily reported slight improvement, but it was always short-lived, and deterioration rapidly followed. There was no period during which Emily was considered to have entered remission or recovery.

In December 1999, Professor West told Emily that she had almost reached the end of the line for treatment of 'intractable' depression. "But," he said, "there is still one final option. Psychosurgery. Brain surgery for psychiatric conditions. Now known as NMD, neurosurgery for mental disorder." He quickly reassured her that the current operation was far more advanced than the frontal lobotomies of the past.

Nothing made sense. How could it have come to this when she had tried everything? ECT and medication contributed to Emily's confusion and having lost sight of what led her to seek help in the first place a long while ago, she had no idea why it had spiralled out of control. She felt like a drop of water being swept along in a rivulet on its way to the sewer.

## PSYCHOSURGERY

Despite being at home for almost all of the school holidays during the intervening years, Emily was aware she had already missed so much of the children's lives. Rachel had moved on to the English National Ballet School, Steve was doing GCSEs, Natalie was now at White Lodge and Harry had just started secondary school. Peter was just about holding it together but plagued by the dread of a phone call to say that Emily was dead. Emily had little agency for her life and the recent failures compounded her sense of futility. She agreed to be referred to the Maudsley Hospital in London for consideration of psychosurgery (NMD) where she was accepted onto their waiting list.

Once again, Emily was sectioned and detained in the DOP. Professor West moved on to a new position and Dr Smith took over, as the new head of the mood disorders service. After six months Emily was still persistently suicidal, the self-harm was risky and dangerous – her section was renewed. The children weren't allowed to visit their mum in hospital and Emily was no longer allowed any visits home. As contact with Peter and the family dwindled, her isolation made it harder for Emily to maintain an interest in their lives; she watched her children grow up from a distance and at the same time grow away from her.

In hospital Emily was irritable and morose; her life was dominated by self-hatred and her mind was filled with a repeating series of strange, bizarre thoughts compelling her to hurt herself on a regular basis. After each act of self-harm, she was taken under duress to A&E and left feeling even worse about herself. Any remnant of self-respect had been trampled on by those paid to care as they made little effort to hide their displeasure and their disdain.

Serena, her therapist, asked the most obvious and logical question. "If you hate the consequences so much, why do you keep doing it?"

Emily didn't know what to say. She felt totally out of control and unable to stop the vicious cycle. She was also petrified that the staff were right. Maybe she didn't want to get better. Maybe she was a fraud.

## SOLUTIONS

The nurses on the ward continued to suggest logical distraction techniques.

She was given an elastic band to flick on her wrist

She was told to go and listen to music

She was told to go and watch TV.

But there was nothing logical about Emily's life, isolated from her loved ones and locked on a psychiatric ward. Inevitably another ghastly trip to A&E followed.

When Dr Smith heard that the Maudsley's programme for NMD had closed, he immediately referred Emily to the only other centre in the UK which performed these drastic operations. In February 2001, Peter accompanied her to Scotland for the assessment by the 'Advanced Interventions Service' (AIS) at Ninewells Hospital in Dundee. AIS was led by Professor Scott, a psychiatrist who was researching novel treatments for psychiatric conditions that had failed to respond to conventional therapies. Henry Scott was a charismatic character, and Emily thought he seemed different from the other psychiatrists she had met. She was impressed by his understanding of her illness. He was kind, compassionate and charming. He didn't judge her for her lack of recovery, nor for her recurrent self-harm.

Professor Scott was passionate about his research and utterly convinced that depression was caused by physical problems in the brain. The proposed experimental surgical intervention (brain surgery) was only offered to patients with severe and intractable (treatment-resistant) depression or more commonly intractable OCD (obsessive-compulsive disorder). All patients had to have had a sufficient trial with the whole gamut of recognised treatments and most patients referred to the AIS left with advice for alternative drug therapies. Only about three patients a year went on to be offered NMD – psychosurgery.

Emily had to complete numerous rating scales of symptom severity for various psychiatric diagnoses, and she was assessed with neuro-cognitive tests using computerised tasks and standardised questions with the team's psychologist. The results painted a pretty gloomy picture. When the full assessment was completed, she was transferred back to the DOP in Southampton with the news that she had met the selection criteria. Emily was offered a place on the research project to undergo an experimental surgical operation called bilateral anterior cingulotomy, to reduce her symptoms. Professor Scott emphasised that this operation was *not curative.*

Emily was still having maintenance ECT and retained little of what she was told in Dundee. The information sheet about the research and NMD was extremely frightening, but she did remember how nice Professor Scott was and she thought she could trust him; he was the only person who instilled a glimmer of hope in her otherwise hopeless situation.

\* \* \*

*Perhaps it was Professor Scott's charismatic personality that won Emily over and secured her consent for such drastic treatment. Psychiatrists tread a difficult path when it comes to working with their vulnerable and disempowered patients. The desire to please can be particularly strong in some people. How is it for you? Do you fully understand the consequences of any treatment that you have assented to? Have you been supported to make independent decisions?*

# CHAPTER 16

# Psychosurgery in Dundee

It was made abundantly clear to all concerned that the proposed experimental brain surgery (NMD) was not curative, and that no realistic improvement in the patient's condition was expected until nine to twelve months after the operation. All patients participating in the research were required to undergo a prolonged period of CBT (Cognitive Behaviour Therapy) after the surgery, to maximise any benefit from the procedure. In Emily's case, the hope was that if successful, she might once again be able to live at home. Her name was put on the waiting list while funding for the procedure was sought from the local clinical commissioners.

In the meantime, Emily's medication was changed to the standardised protocol for treatment-resistant depression patients participating in the Dundee research. She was already taking sertraline, olanzapine, mirtazapine, lithium, sodium valproate, chlorpromazine and nitrazepam. The sertraline was stopped and replaced with unlicensed, high-dose venlafaxine at 600mg. In March, ketoconazole, another 'adjuvant' drug, was added to the bizarre cocktail of drugs.

## MAYFLOWER

Before long, Emily lost the transient ray of hope the visit to Dundee had given her. The nurses on the ward lost patience with her and simultaneously a doctor from A&E sent a letter warning the psychiatric team that Emily was at high risk of death if the self-harm continued. By this time Emily had become a notorious 'frequent attender', although she never gave the A&E staff any trouble when she was taken there for treatment. Rather, she was like a sad, little mouse unable to say boo to a goose. Dr Smith transferred Emily to the psychiatric intensive care unit (Mayflower), where she would be observed more closely, to be 'kept safe' until they could get her to Scotland for the surgery.

The entrance to Mayflower ward was through a double set of doors separated by an air lock, ensuring that there was no escape. Children were prohibited from visiting and even visits from Peter were strictly controlled. As days went by, Emily became less and less convinced that she wanted to go through with the NMD. When one of the other patients had managed to die by suicide despite being locked up in Mayflower ward – this high security unit – Emily learned how he did it. She took her chance – and failed. It ensured she was placed on 'suicide watch', twenty-four-hour surveillance where she was never left alone, and it continued for the next few months. A nurse was stationed with her inside the small single room, and she lost all rights to privacy, even in the toilet and bathroom. As a further disincentive to curtail any further self-harming behaviour, Emily was banned from having any visitors.

Though the stakes had been raised, she wasn't ready to give in. One night, the nurse sitting on a chair at the end of her bed fell asleep. Emily made as little movement as possible as she reached under the bed-frame to the blade sellotaped beneath the mattress. Her cut wasn't as deep as she wanted before the nurse woke to see the crimson colour of blood seeping through the blanket. Everyone was angry with her and from that time on, they insisted that both her hands must be visible at all times, including through the night. She was woken repeatedly if her hands slipped out of sight beneath the sheets.

## FAREWELL

News came that funding had been agreed for the surgery and a date was set for her transfer to Dundee in September 2001. Peter asked if he might be allowed to take Emily out for a couple of hours to watch their youngest son, Harry, who been chosen as a mascot for the Southampton football team in their new stadium. Permission was granted only on condition that Emily made no further attempts to self-harm; it sealed her compliance. This was successful and she earned one final concession before the journey to Scotland. Peter was allowed to take her out to a local restaurant, to join all the family for Rachel's farewell. Rachel had graduated from ballet school and was leaving to take up her first job as a professional ballet dancer.

Two trained nurses escorted Emily the six-hundred-mile journey to the Carseview Centre, the inpatient psychiatric unit, adjacent to Ninewells Hospital in Dundee, where her brain surgery was due to take place. Before the operation Emily completed another battery of rating scales and was videoed during a standardised interview for the research. Her case would be scrutinised by an independent committee to confirm her suitability for the procedure and verify her consent. Before she met with them, it was explained to her the surgery could not take place without their ratification. Written reports were also submitted to the committee from members of the psychiatric team, and included a statement that her prognosis was so poor that she would likely die if the surgery did not go ahead. Emily had her own secret reason for wanting the operation. She had decided that her family must know that she had tried every possible option before she killed herself.

## BRAIN SURGERY

A few days after the surgery, her face was swollen from the leak of CSF (cerebrospinal fluid) from around her brain, into the tissues. She had a fever and a terrible headache. Professor Scott sighed in frustration when Emily asked exactly what operation she had had. Despite her supposed consent, the only thing Emily had remembered being told was that it wouldn't change her personality.

He explained she had undergone a 'bilateral anterior cingulotomy', an apparently low-risk, stereotactic procedure where the neurosurgeon placed small electrodes in an area of the brain called the cingulate gyrus under MRI guidance. An electric current heated the tips of these electrodes, so that they destroyed an area of brain tissue about the size of a pea on both sides of the anterior cingulate. This meant very little to Emily as she had no idea what these parts of the brain were supposed to do.

Professor Scott and his team had no concrete theories about why this surgery apparently helped some patients but not others. Since there was no expectation of immediate improvement after the surgery, the post-operative focus was on making sure the patients followed a standardised plan, by continuing the set regime of prescribed drugs and participating in regular CBT for one year.

Each patient was set a predetermined goal which would help define whether they were a 'responder' or not for the purposes of the research. If Emily was well enough to be discharged from hospital and that was maintained for a year, it would be regarded as a 'successful outcome'. Any return to work as a doctor was completely out of the question.

Emily was still on strict twenty-four-hour observation and confined to one room on September 11th 2001. She had no access to a TV or a radio. She heard people talking excitedly in the corridor outside her room but knew nothing of the catastrophic events in America that day. Having been detained on a locked psychiatric ward for over a year, she was completely oblivious to what was going on in the world outside.

## FATAL DECISION

Once Emily's physical recovery from the surgery was well under way, Professor Scott explained what the next steps would be. Once she was fit enough to return to Southampton, it had been decided that it was no longer reasonable to keep her confined on the psychiatric intensive care unit. She would still be detained under the Mental Health Act and would still remain under lock and key, but on a completely different ward at the DOP, where she had never been previously. Emily wanted to know why. Professor Scott was honest as he spelled it out to her. The nursing staff on her previous ward did not want her back, stating that their relationship with Emily had completely broken down.

This was the straw that broke the camel's back. Faced with the strength of the animosity towards her, this final humiliation was enough to seal Emily's fate. She had no doubts now that she must find a way to kill herself. Still on twenty-four-hour suicide watch, Emily spent the next few days quietly trying to devise a plan. She made a pact with herself: no more failed attempts.

After the surgery, Emily's drug regime had been drastically changed. All her previous five drugs had been stopped except the venlafaxine which had been reduced from 600mg to 375mg, and mirtazapine was also reduced down to 45mg. (Zopiclone was continued for sleep.)

## MIRACLE

It was Friday evening, eight days after the surgery, when a nurse accompanied Emily to a small sitting room, allowed to watch TV. Another patient came in complaining, "All I want, is to be at home with my husband and children." She remembers momentary irritation, when suddenly without warning, a light switched on in her head. It felt like a tangible physical sensation as if the power cables of a generator had been connected. Her next thought echoed that of the annoying patient. *All I want, is to be at home with my husband and children*, and she cried for the first time in years. She had no idea what had just happened, but she knew it was remarkable and she also knew the depression was over. A loud thought almost like a voice followed. *What about the self-harm?* Emily was determined as she said back to it, *I don't want that anymore.*

That same internal dialogue repeated itself over the next couple of days and then it stopped.

The nurse guarding Emily was sitting beside her and didn't appear to notice the tears. Emily didn't dare tell anyone what had happened because she needed to be absolutely sure it was real. She didn't tell Peter when he called that evening. He was due to fly up to Scotland on Sunday and stay in Dundee until Emily was ready to be transferred back to Southampton, tasked with the responsibility of accompanying her for the journey. When he arrived two days later, he was immediately struck by the change in her demeanour. Emily was beaming, delighted to see him and finally she was ready to tell someone what had happened. Naturally it was good that Peter was the first to hear her describe her light experience and that the sense of well-being had continued.

Peter, in turn, somewhat tentatively, decided to share what had been going on behind the scenes at home. A group of Christians from around the Southampton region had been meeting regularly to pray specifically for Emily's recovery. Peter had been reluctant to tell her because she had become so antagonistic to any mention of healing prayer. Now it seemed obvious to both of them – the light experience was a miracle.

## SCEPTICISM

After the weekend, Professor Scott invited Peter and Emily into one of the interview rooms for a chat. Emily confidently related the light experience to him, explaining that she felt completely better. Sitting opposite her, Professor Scott frowned. This had not happened to any other patients. He thought it was probably a placebo response and cautioned Peter and Emily not to read too much into it. But his face lightened up as he suggested that Peter take Emily out for the rest of the day.

It was cold and windy, but they didn't mind. For the next few days, they felt like regular holidaymakers as Emily was granted further leave, only returning to the ward to stay overnight. They met Rachel at the airport – she had a couple of days leave from the ballet company and it was a delightful reunion. Emily reflected on how thoughtful and encouraging Rachel had been throughout the whole ordeal, sending her little notes when she wasn't able to see her. It was an emotional farewell when the time came for Rachel's departure back to Germany.

Perhaps Professor Scott's scepticism on Emily's progress was increased by the fact that her scores on all the depression rating scales were worse than before the surgery. She tried to explain to him that the questions were not clear enough to accurately reflect how she was feeling since the light experience. Indeed, she had felt worse immediately after the operation. The only evidence of Emily's improvement, for the research, was the change in her demeanour recorded on video when they repeated the standardised interview.

## SECURITY

Professor Scott came to say goodbye to Peter and Emily just before they left for Southampton. He was pleased that she still felt better but warned them again that it was highly likely her depressive symptoms would return. He reminded her that she must continue all the drugs for at least a year, as well as engage with CBT.

Emily was buoyant and dismissed his concerns. Professor Scott agreed to sanction a 'transgression', to allow Peter to take Emily home for supper – strictly speaking, she was supposed to be taken straight to the DOP from the airport. But first Emily had to discover how the world had moved on in a very practical way with the adoption of new security measures for air travel.

It was her coat having to go through the X-ray machine that alarmed Emily the most. She breathed a sigh of relief that she wasn't stopped. Before travelling to Scotland for the surgery, Emily had hidden a blade in the coat lining, but had been unable to find it once she arrived on the ward in Dundee. There was a lot of catching up to do.

On the home front, Emily was surprised to learn that their daughter Natalie had left the Royal Ballet School. Peter was driving her back to White Lodge after a weekend home when she had burst into tears, saying she didn't want to go back. Peter turned the car round and took her back home. Even after a period of recuperation and pleas from White Lodge for this talented dancer to return, Natalie remained firm about her decision. Peter honoured their promise not to make her stay if she changed her mind, and so she joined her younger brother at the local comprehensive.

Emily had not set foot in her home for over a year and was bowled over by how much the children had grown up. Natalie had a meal ready and waiting for them, the boys helped out and Emily was overwhelmed by the desire to come home and stay home. But she was still detained on a section and Peter was legally bound to return her to the DOP. By the time they drove into the hospital car park, Emily was utterly distraught. It felt just like going back to boarding school. Peter did his best to comfort her, begging her to hang on. They couldn't afford her tears to be misinterpreted as a sign she was still depressed. Once she managed to regain her composure, reluctantly, they climbed the stairs and rang the bell to be admitted to the new ward.

## ASTONISHMENT

The following morning, Dr Smith could not conceal his astonishment when he saw Emily. He had received updates from Dundee, but he conceded she was a totally different person. He remained cautious but allowed Emily to go home for the day. After only two nights on the ward, Dr Smith authorised Emily's home leave, conditional upon attending the ward for a daily review by a member of his team. Technically, Dr Smith still had the power to recall her to hospital at any time if he determined it necessary. It took a few weeks to reassure himself that Emily's recovery was authentic and then he officially discharged her from both the section and the hospital.

How fantastic it would have been if the story had ended there. None of the psychiatrists had any explanation for Emily's remarkable recovery. Did the radical reduction in her drug regimen post-operatively play any part in this sudden return to normality?

Emily thought that God had healed her, and it would be over forever. Sadly, she was wrong; the psychiatrists were expecting relapse, and they were right for the wrong reasons. The root causes of her original crisis remained unresolved. There was more to come before she would finally be released from the shackles of life as a psychiatric patient.

\* \* \*

*Maybe this parallels your own experiences. It is so disappointing when better times do not last, but please do not give up hope. Is it possible that traumatic events from your past need further attention to sustain recovery? Can you think of any other reasons why you may be feeling less well right now?*

# CHAPTER 17

# The psychiatrist's summary

It is staggering to think what Emily and her family went through during those extraordinarily long and painful seven years. All because she did what she thought was right and sought help from her doctor.

The psychiatrists reassured Emily that her memory loss resulting from ECT was a good thing, but her body did not forget. Whenever she was in the vicinity of the hospitals where she had been admitted, it triggered a fight, flight or freeze response.

## REBELLION

Despite the advice to continue her antidepressants for at least a year, Emily wasn't happy. She hated being overweight and she hated her clothes, like the cheap 'old lady' trousers with elasticated waists a relative had given her while her weight kept going up at an alarming rate. She was sure mirtazapine was responsible for her abnormally voracious appetite and she suspected it was also causing her daytime lethargy. The time had come when she was no longer willing to put up with the unpleasant adverse effects that had plagued her for years and so she stopped taking mirtazapine.

What she didn't know was that stopping psychiatric drugs abruptly could lead to withdrawal. But she was still taking venlafaxine, and she didn't notice any difference, except how rewarding it was to feel more alert. She started to diet and exercise in an attempt to bring her weight down to her previous normal. The next drug she stopped was zopiclone. This was definitely more of a challenge, and for nights on end she couldn't sleep due to the severe rebound insomnia.

When Emily was reviewed in outpatients, she was honest about what she had done but determined not to complain of any symptoms. The psychiatrists were still not fully convinced that she was recovered and while their expectations for her relapse were high, she had no desire to trigger any suspicions in their minds. Dr Smith was very insistent that she continue to take venlafaxine at least until the anniversary of the surgery.

## SUMMARISING SEVEN YEARS

Dr Smith's team were preparing a presentation on Emily's case for fellow psychiatrists and invited Peter and Emily to come and answer questions. They formulated a timeline from December 1994 to October 2001 which summarised all the major events including all Emily's admissions, and treatments, including the drug changes, ECT and even the prescribed sleep deprivation therapy. The conclusion was that it had been one single episode of intractable, treatment-resistant depression lasting a total of six years, and ten months.

Today, the detail of the summary is still astonishing and in retrospect, it is difficult to comprehend just how many drugs Emily was prescribed over that period of time and the extreme treatments which she endured. Yet this happened with the intention of ending Emily's suffering, while her psychiatrists believed she had an unusually severe, treatment-resistant depression. Emily was prescribed thirty-three different drugs specifically to treat her depression, during the time period from her first visit to the GP to the current day. These included various different 'classes' of psychiatric drugs. (For further detail and explanation, see appendix.)

- 14 antidepressants including SSRIs, SNRIs, MAOIs, Tricyclics, other non-classified.
- 9 antipsychotics including 'older' neuroleptics and depot injections, newer types.
- 2 mood stabilisers including lithium.
- 3 'adjunct' drugs for intractable depression.
- 5 benzodiazepine & Z-drugs.
- Total = 33.

And three further psychoactive drugs to treat side effects:

- 1 anti-Parkinson's drug (for tremor).
- 2 antiemetic drugs (for nausea).
- Final Total = 36.

In addition to modifying the complex array of different combinations of these drugs, the doses were frequently increased. Sometimes a drug was stopped only to be reintroduced at a later date and Emily would be prescribed other drugs purely to treat the adverse effects of those which were supposed to be treating the depression. (Not listed above.) But none of this 'treatment' made Emily any better. In fact, she suffered a huge number of adverse effects (side effects), some of which resulted in significant illness or injury. These included:

- Postural hypotension – Emily fainted and required sutures to her head.

- Permanent hypothyroidism secondary to lithium – requiring treatment with levothyroxine.
- Amenorrhoea – her periods stopped, leading to osteopenia (bone thinning), requiring treatment with Vitamin D and calcium supplements.
- Weight gain and obesity.
- Oversedation leading to unsteadiness. She fell and suffered a serious head injury which gave her double vision. Emily needed a CT and a referral to neurology. She was diagnosed with a sixth nerve palsy. Thankfully this recovered spontaneously.
- Hyperprolactinaemia – raised levels of the hormone prolactin.
- Low hormone levels of cortisol.
- Nausea – requiring antiemetics.
- Parkinsonian symptoms – tremor, rigidity – treatment with procyclidine.
- Constipation – laxatives.
- Dry mouth and difficulty swallowing.
- Recurrent choking led to more investigations and another drug – prescribed to treat the erratic oesophageal contractions which were evident on a 'barium swallow'. This fully recovered only after psychiatric medications were stopped.

The other symptoms which could have been attributable to adverse effects of her psychiatric medications but were always taken to be symptoms of depression:

- Self-harm and suicidality.
- Feeling numb, unable to experience emotion.
- Feelings of unreality.
- Depersonalisation – feeling outside herself.
- Auditory hallucinations – hearing voices.

- Stupor, lethargy, loss of energy, fatigue.
- Severe sleep disturbance – insomnia alternating with hypersomnia (sleeping too much).
- Agitation/akathisia – constant restlessness that caused Emily great distress and led her to pace up and down.
- Restless leg syndrome – restlessness confined to the legs, often at night.
- Severe sexual dysfunction – unable to have an enjoyable sex life.

## ECT SUMMARY

Emily endured over one hundred ECT treatments, sometimes without consent, when mandated on a section. After ECT treatments, she was often profoundly disorientated and confused, as well as having a severe headache. Emily suffered permanent memory loss for some significant events around the periods when she had ECT. This included her sister's wedding and Rachel's graduation performance of *Les Sylphides* where she performed the starring role at the end of her ballet training. Both memories have been completely erased. To this day, even though Emily knows she was present; it feels as though she was never there.

Jean, a fellow patient who contacted Emily years after the event, describes how she used to sit there "in another world" after ECT. Jean said it heavily influenced her own decision to refuse to undergo ECT.

Emily also experienced:

1. Anaesthetic complication as a result of a rare genetic disorder (pseudocholinesterase deficiency aka suxamethonium apnoea); her breathing had to be maintained by 'bag-mask ventilation' for twenty minutes.
2. Awake paralysis during ECT.

3. 'Slow to wake up' after ECT – which prompted further investigations including CT scan.
4. 'Slow to respond' – which led to multiple treatments and then 'maintenance ECT'.

## EXTREME TREATMENT

After all these treatments failed, Emily was subjected to permanent, irreversible, experimental brain surgery, where healthy brain tissue was destroyed.

I doubt that the facts of Emily's case were presented in this way. Peter and Emily were asked to wait outside until the presentation was finished before they were invited into the room to answer questions. There was silence. Eventually one of the psychiatrists asked Emily, "Why did you deliberately self-harm?"

It took her by surprise and all she could remember was how derogatory staff had been and she felt very uncomfortable. Her reply was defensive: "I wasn't trying to seek attention."

There were no more questions and no further opportunity for these expert psychiatrists to learn from Emily and Peter's experience. She felt like a curiosity being displayed at a fair.

## EMILY'S REFLECTION

It took time and considerable courage before Emily was ready to really think through and reflect on what had happened over the last seven years. When she saw herself in the mirror and looked at her tremendously scarred abdomen, Emily wanted to face up to the reasons why she had behaved in such uncharacteristic ways. She hardly recognised herself. She thought she really must have been crazy.

Most of the psychiatrists and the community psychiatric nurses had shown considerable compassion when treating

Emily. There were also some excellent, kind and caring nurses when she was in hospital, and she wanted all of them to know how much she appreciated their outstanding efforts to help her. Nonetheless, she still had terrible memories from her repeated incarcerations on locked psychiatric wards where some of the nurses had been very unkind, antagonistic or who had lost patience with her; she had also witnessed similar punitive attitudes towards fellow patients, some of whom remain friends to this present day. Emily could not readily forget the cruel treatment in A&E by cynical and jaded staff.

## LAWYER

While she sought to understand her own behaviour, she found the recollections of what had happened incredibly painful. She thought she should hold the NHS to account for the abuse she had suffered and seek legal redress, if only to stop it happening to other people. But when she finally found a medical negligence lawyer who was willing to listen to her, she was disappointed. His assessment was blunt. He said she would not stand a chance in a million of winning her case. He said the courts would put more weight on the opinions given by those very staff who needed to answer for their actions.

"They will scrutinise in detail every entry in your medical record. Do you really want them to hear the hospital staff's denials of any allegations you make? Do you really want your personal life and that of your family to be dissected in the public arena of a court? You were detained because they assessed you as being a danger to yourself, why would they believe what you have to say? Wouldn't they rather favour the words of the 'dedicated' doctors and nurses who cared for you? They would wipe the floor with you."

When Emily remembered how her one letter of complaint had backfired, she realised it was indeed futile. In short, there was no way that she could prove that she had been harmed. Though Emily wrestled with the injustice, she had to let it go.

## EXPERTS

Emily noticed that now she was recovered, her psychiatrists treated her with the kind of respect given to fellow medical colleagues. Both the professors, Scott and West, as well as Dr Smith, reiterated how unusual she was in being so ill with a severe, treatment-resistant depression. Professor West went further, telling her he had never come across such a serious case of depression as Emily's in his career. They weren't entirely sure what caused her brain to malfunction, but they were sure her depression was endogenous, meaning it was caused by a biological problem, and was not a reaction to circumstances. They still talked vaguely about chemical imbalance.

Emily had always assumed that scientific research evidenced the theories of psychiatric diagnosis, drug treatments and ECT. Of course, she knew the neurosurgery was still experimental, but Professor Scott was very enthusiastic about its benefits and convinced that it was only a matter of time before the 'real and correctable abnormalities' would be found. When they talked to her, she was mesmerised by their expertise and felt indebted to them because they never gave up on her. Emily repeatedly asked what they thought had happened to explain her apparent miraculous recovery, but none of them had any answers.

## CBT

Undoubtedly the years as a psychiatric patient had been an extreme test of endurance, but Emily was motivated to believe that somehow it had to have been worth it in the end. At least she could console herself that she had proved the cynics and sceptics wrong. She had always wanted to get better and now, here she was, fully recovered.

Ironically, it was the CBT therapist (Tracy) who predicted the future with the most accuracy. At the first appointment, Emily had no symptoms of depression and Tracy seemed uncertain about how to proceed. She didn't seem impressed with Emily's recovery and asked Emily to do some homework prior to the next session. But Emily was irritated by the request to write down how she coped with negative experiences during the week. She thought she'd had more than enough trouble and didn't want to focus on the negative. Tracy rebuked her sharply. "You have fallen off the horse once, don't think it won't happen again."

Perhaps if Tracy had been more empathic, Emily would not have cancelled her next appointment, because actually Tracy was right; nothing had changed and the original reasons for the emotional crisis back in 1994 were still unresolved. But Emily didn't know that it was her childhood survival persona which programmed the way she reacted to stress, and she had no role models to teach her self-care.

While Emily's psychiatrists remained convinced that her childhood traumas had not caused her depression, she felt duty-bound to try and forget about the past. Of course, she had no insight into the fact that her admissions to psychiatric institutions bore remarkable similarities to her boarding school experiences and had effectively re-traumatised her.

\* \* \*

*What is your experience of being treated with therapy, psychiatric drugs or ECT? Have you been treated with multiple medications? What is your conclusion about the effectiveness of any treatment you have received? Have you any side effects that are bothering you? There are plenty of people with lived experience who have found different ways of recovery. The websites Mad In the UK and Mad In America are useful resources to look at the alternatives (details in Appendix).*

# CHAPTER 18

# Homecoming

Emily's homecoming was a celebration of triumph over adversity and the whole family assumed that their collective nightmare was over. She sang worship songs out loud as she unpacked her suitcase to put her clothes away in her own bedroom drawers and relished the moment as she placed her toothbrush in the cup in the bathroom which held four others. Simple freedoms like being able to eat and drink whatever she wanted at any time of the day and night felt delightful. She took her time as she ambled down the road, past the small front gardens of the neighbouring houses, struck by the familiarity of it all.

While appreciating her liberty, she was like a soldier returned from war in the discovery that her family had moved on without her. Emily was proud at the way they managed but she had barely seen them over the last year, and she overestimated their recovery. As she tried to re-establish herself as part of the family, she made many mistakes. All four of the children had learnt to carry on without her and it was a major readjustment for them to accommodate their mum back into their lives. Aware that she had missed out on so much, Emily badly wanted to make it up to them. Emily was in a rush and knew little about how her adolescent children ticked.

Rachel had left home completely and was now settled in Germany as a professional ballet dancer. The other three children attended local secondary schools and were not used to having Mum around 'interfering' with their independence.

## REALITY

The initial euphoria was short-lived. Emily was desperate to catch up, yet it was taboo to speak of what she had been through. Perhaps it was a similar story when someone returns home, having served time in prison. Home life was difficult and stressful for all of them and the repercussions from this period in their lives were deep and prolonged. Peter and Emily were trying hard to re-establish their marriage relationship. Peter was utterly exhausted, and Emily couldn't understand why he didn't appear happier now it was all over. It would take time to reshape and restore the previous intimacy of a loving marriage. It must have been extremely difficult for the children to see their parents in turmoil. Neither friends, relatives, nor professionals had the foresight to understand that the family couldn't just switch back to 'normality'. Now she was well, all Emily's support had been withdrawn.

## PERSPECTIVE

Over a decade later in Denver, when Barb shared her insights, she surmised that while the children were young, they had seen their mother as 'the strong doctor' which changed suddenly when she became ill. They would have experienced terrible anxiety and uncertainty over their mum's welfare. It was irrelevant that Emily had always wanted to be a good mother and had always intended to be there for them. Neither did it matter that she never wanted the children to get hurt. Emily could never rectify the pain her children suffered during her erratic and repeated absences during the hospital admissions. Barb said that each of her four children would have had their own individual, unspoken, unrealistic, and unattainable expectations of what she would be like. There was a disparity between the mum of their hopes and dreams and the one who returned and who didn't live up to their picture of who she should be.

Members of the wider family, many of whom Emily hadn't spoken to in years, started to get in touch. Other friends and family who had become accustomed to seeing Emily as an invalid, also had some difficulty readjusting to Emily's sudden bounce back to health. Though Emily knew they meant well, she hated being the focus of their worry.

"Are you sure you can manage?"

"Don't you think you need a little rest now?"

However much she tried to reassure them that she was not ungrateful, inevitably it caused a certain amount of tension when she insisted on reasserting her independence.

## CHURCH PROPHECY

Since the psychiatrists could not give an explanation for Emily's light experience and recovery, both Peter and Emily remained convinced that God had intervened in a miraculous way. Now Emily believed she had been healed, she thought it was time to take God seriously again and it wasn't long before she returned to the very heart of the charismatic Christian scene.

Emily was invited to tell her story to a packed congregation of around six hundred people at church. The preacher for that day referred back to what Emily had shared during his sermon, and then addressed her directly. "You have had seven years of curses, but now you will have seven years filled with blessings."

He elaborated further, saying that God was going to use Emily to heal others, and the church applauded. After the service, the congregation gathered around the large hall area to have coffee, and a few friendships were renewed. One person even apologised for losing contact because of her illness, explaining that they just couldn't cope. Peter and Emily went home on a high, buoyed up by the fact that God hadn't forgotten them.

It was hard when Emily found herself being asked to pray for a lady who had terminal cancer. Reluctantly she agreed to visit Rose at home, but only after explaining that her healing had nothing to do with her own level of faith; in fact, she had given up on God and given up on prayer. As they sat and talked, Rose asked, "Why did you and your family have to suffer for so long, if God was going to heal you anyway?"

This was a very legitimate question and Emily had no answer. She was the antithesis of a healer and couldn't square the circle. Tragically Rose died. Within a year two young men, also associated with the church community, died by suicide. It left Emily feeling angry as well as perplexed. *How could God heal me but not them?* None of it made sense and then there was another shock to come.

News broke that one of Natalie's friends had been abducted, raped, and murdered a couple of miles from where they lived. The following Sunday at church, Emily sat with her arms around Natalie, both of them in tears. It seemed totally incomprehensible, and Emily wondered how God could possibly allow this to happen. After the service was over, someone came over and whispered in Emily's ear, "I'm so sorry to see that you're depressed again."

Emily was appalled. She was grieving for a young girl who had just lost her life in tragic circumstances, and yet some ignoramus didn't think twice about slapping a depression sticker right back on her forehead.

## TURBULENCE

Emily had to find a way to harness her growing sense of frustration. She deep-cleaned the house from top to bottom, which was badly needed after years of neglect. She cleared out her wardrobe and threw away everything that could possibly remind her of the nightmare years. She was determined to completely redecorate the house and seriously thought about moving, even getting to the stage of contacting estate agents.

It remained a turbulent period in their lives and Emily was conscious of the way she remained under everyone's gaze. If she mentioned problems, she noticed the subtle changes in expression which registered suspicion. It felt as if her mental health was public property, and she resented their negative expectations when they thought she was not out of the woods. She hated the way people asked whether she still took medication, always wrapped in a veneer of concern. It wasn't anyone else's business, but Emily lacked the skills to deal with it assertively. Instead, she reverted to the survival persona of the past and became more guarded, internalising her feelings.

## OTHER ALLEGIANCES

On one occasion, Emily sought help from a friend who also had older teens. Jill welcomed Emily into her beautiful, colour-coordinated living room. Emily looked round, admiring the tasteful décor, thinking how neglected her own house looked now. Jill joined her with a pot of tea and Emily leant forwards from her comfortable seat on the sofa to describe a particular challenge with one of her children. "You handled it completely wrong," Jill replied. The chastisement continued as she expanded on Emily's faulty parenting. Suddenly the penny dropped as Emily realised that Jill already knew all about the situation. Of course! She would always be grateful that Jill was a natural confidante to her child when she wasn't around, but she left her house, smarting.

On the walk home, the world didn't appear so bright or colourful anymore and Emily was horrified by her failure as a mother. As she passed the closed doors and shut windows of houses in the neighbourhood, all of a sudden, she felt cold, not knowing who she could confide in or where she could find help in the future. Perhaps their deficiencies as parents were already common knowledge within their relatively small social circle of church friends. Emily felt both guilty and ashamed. Her emotions were in danger of spiralling out of control and once again, she retreated and battened down the hatches, terrified of being labelled as depressed again. None of this helped her adolescent children.

They had wanted to do the right thing when Peter and Emily had arranged for private counselling for one of the children; bizarrely, the counsellor paid them a visit and also heaped further criticism on their heads. It seemed that wherever they looked for help, people were all too willing to tell them how badly they were doing, yet unable to approach their extraordinary situation constructively or with compassion.

Meanwhile, the pressure on Peter and Emily's marriage was increasing. They were on the brink of separation when thankfully, they managed to pause and step back. They had been good together before Emily's illness, even though they hadn't always communicated as fully as they should have done. Peter was a very kind and thoughtful man. Emily knew that he had sacrificed everything to do the best for their family. He was a good father. They had no qualms over admitting they had made mistakes and they recognised how well they had done in getting through the whole ordeal. Peter and Emily made up their differences and buried the hatchet. This was the breakthrough that was needed and at last life at home started to become slightly easier.

## VENLAFAXINE WITHDRAWAL

In outpatients, Dr Smith encouraged Emily to get on with her life, and she wanted to discharge herself from any more follow-up feeling that it was completely unnecessary. She was now absolutely sure that venlafaxine was causing the continued sexual dysfunction and was not prepared to put up with it any longer. But it was too embarrassing to discuss with Dr Smith. She didn't want to tell him that she planned to stop the venlafaxine, especially as she still needed his support both for the reinstatement of her driving licence and to return to work.

Knowing nothing about withdrawal, Emily was very alarmed when she started to experience weird and unpleasant electric-shock-like sensations going all through her body. Reluctantly she gave Dr Smith a call and admitted that she had reduced the dose of venlafaxine as she was going to stop it. He seemed to understand her reasoning and said he'd heard of other patients experiencing similar effects, so at least she knew she wasn't going crazy. But Dr Smith wasn't any the wiser about how to overcome these symptoms; his only advice was to lower the dose very slowly.

Through trial and error, Emily found her own way of dealing with it; she reverted back to a slightly higher dose and then tried much longer intervals before attempting a further dose reduction. The venlafaxine came in capsules, and she found that the only way to do this was to open them up and divide the tiny little beads into smaller and smaller portions, strung over weeks. When she was down to a very tiny amount, she only took it when the unpleasant shocks became intolerable, all the while slowly lengthening the period in between each dose.

Emily had broken her promise to continue the antidepressants for at least a year, but she was very happy to have her sex life back and triumphant to have stopped all her psychiatric drugs. Furthermore, she felt back to her normal self and had no symptoms which could be labelled as depression.

## MOVING FORWARDS

Determined to leave the sick-role behind, Emily informed the benefits office of her recovery, explaining that she no longer required 'incapacity benefit'. A couple of weeks later, Peter received a letter from the benefits office, offering their condolences making an assumption that she had died. Emily found it hilarious and called them back to say that on the contrary, she was very much alive!

The thwarted attempt to return to work a few years earlier stood Emily in good stead. Armed with clearance from occupational health and her psychiatrist's blessing, she obtained an honorary contract to start work as an unpaid clinical observer in A&E at Southampton General Hospital.

Admittedly it was a nerve-wracking prospect to return to the department where she had attended as a patient so frequently during the previous year. As she walked up the hill to the hospital for her first shift, she repeatedly told herself: "It was not my fault I was depressed. I self-harmed because I was ill. I am well, this is the real me, back in my right mind." She was relieved that few people in A&E recognised her, but she had rehearsed what to say, just in case they did.

After a couple of weeks, one of the consultants asked if she would cover a shift as a locum. She was thrilled to be paid for the first time in almost eight years and help reverse the debt, which had meant they couldn't afford a holiday that year.

Better still, Emily was accepted back onto the flexible training scheme that she had never quite managed to start. On 1st August 2002, she commenced her part-time postgraduate training as a senior house officer (SHO) in Emergency Medicine, exactly seven and a half years later than originally scheduled.

It was unfortunate that Peter's company sent him to work in the Bahamas on an important project just at the same time that Emily returned to work. He was due to be away for six weeks and as a surprise, Emily decided to completely redecorate their bedroom. Admittedly, it was an ambitious project to attempt on her own and she needed help to dismantle the big white Formica wall unit, a monstrosity left by the previous owner. Emily borrowed a circular saw, to cut it up into manageable chunks which she could then take to the tip in the car. About four weeks into the endeavour, she discovered crumbling plaster beneath the many layers of wallpaper and then the phone rang. It was Peter. "Good news," he said, "the project's finished early, I'll be home in a couple of days."

Emily tried to sound enthusiastic despite her internal panic. It was mayhem. Their bedroom was a complete mess, all the remaining furniture and their belongings had been redistributed to any available space throughout the house. She made a valiant attempt to restore some order before Peter arrived home. He laughed as she showed him their derelict bedroom and willingly agreed to be roped in when really what he needed was a well-earned rest. Peter and Emily were not in the least bit expert when it came to DIY, but they were at their best as they worked together to get it all finished. Since Emily's recovery, it seemed like they had lurched from one calamity to the next, but once more, things were good between them.

\* \* \*

*It was assumed that Emily's husband and children would cope with the transition, and their welfare as a family was never seriously considered. Do you feel that you have the right amount of independence? Have you experienced personalised care which is flexible, responsive, and compassionate? Have you and your family been given all the support you need?*

# CHAPTER 19

# Passion for anti-stigma

Doctors who choose A&E (also known as Emergency Medicine) as a career are attracted by the prospect of becoming experts at treating patients after major trauma or resuscitating those with life-threatening or serious physical illness. Treating patients with mental health problems or self-harm in A&E, was seen as unavoidable but undesirable, almost as if superfluous to their specialised skills. When Emily witnessed the familiar eye-rolling and the same sort of derogatory comments that she had experienced herself, she volunteered to see these patients.

Anti-stigma was already Emily's passion, and she became more determined to teach her colleagues how to understand their psychiatric patients better, abolish punitive attitudes and eliminate discrimination, rudeness, and disrespect. Since psychiatry was always the least popular part of the curriculum, her colleagues were delighted that Emily took it on herself to do the departmental teaching on the subject.

# TEACHER

All Emily knew about psychiatry was what she had been taught at medical school and experienced during her time as a patient. She had never heard anyone doubt the traditional biomedical model of psychiatry, centred on genetics, theories around chemical imbalance and possible structural abnormalities within the brain. Psychiatric conditions were believed to be treatable with drugs; diagnoses such as anxiety, depression, OCD, bipolar and schizophrenia were firmly established in mainstream practice alongside the heavy marketing of psychotropic drugs to treat them.

What Emily did not know was that despite decades of funding ploughed into research there have been no consistent findings to prove the theories. There were genetic studies, MRI studies, molecular studies, and a plethora of drug trials, none of which conclusively validated the existence of specific psychiatric diagnoses. Likewise, there is no convincing evidence that either drugs or ECT could cure these putative conditions.

However, what she set out to do was to challenge people's attitudes. Tentatively at first, Emily began to share her own experiences, describing something of her nightmare 'when seriously ill with treatment-resistant depression' – still fully embracing the narrative spelt out by the psychiatrists. While they conceded that her childhood adversities had given her 'vulnerability factors' for depression, they were adamant they had not caused her depression. Portraying her illness as a 'biological condition' gave her the confidence to share that she had self-harmed with sceptical colleagues.

Admittedly it wasn't easy, she didn't blush, and she didn't look away, but inside she felt herself shrinking. Even with the knowledge, that she could not be responsible for having a 'biological' condition, how could she fully excuse herself when familiar feelings of humiliation bubbled to the surface? The gate had not shut on the well-worn path of self-blame. But Emily was a pro when it came to hiding her feelings and she was on a roll, going from strength to strength.

It seemed obvious to Emily that if the basis of mental illness was chemical imbalance, then patients given the right diagnosis and the right drug treatment would get better. Of course, in medicine there are always exceptions, but Emily had been repeatedly told that it was rare to be like her with such a serious depression that is completely unresponsive to treatment. It made perfect sense therefore, to make sure that patients were referred to psychiatric care in a timely manner to get the treatment they so evidently needed. Emily's colleagues were absolutely delighted that she took such an interest in these patients, and it was not unusual to hear, "Emily, this one's *definitely* for you."

Whenever Emily saw patients with new or established psychiatric diagnoses, she assured them that if they followed their doctor's advice and took their medication, they would soon be better. But Emily discovered there was one well-recognised exception to the rule – psychiatrists had a 'get out of jail free' card and this was in the case of personality disorder. The traditional teaching was that these patients, who had often suffered terrible abuse in childhood, were not amenable to treatment. It was hard to know how to help them, but Emily thought, the very least they could do was be kind and respectful to all patients regardless of their diagnoses.

However, Emily acknowledged that sometimes, some patients with mental health problems who came to A&E were pretty challenging, and she found it puzzling. It was easy enough to fall into the trap of feeling irritated when all she was doing was trying to help. It was early days, and Emily still had a lot to learn.

## PROMOTION

Determined to pursue a career in Emergency Medicine (A&E), Emily passed her postgraduate exams and applied for promotion to Specialist Registrar (SpR) on the local training scheme. Candidates were advised to visit all participating hospitals' A&E's prior to the interviews. There was another doctor also short-listed who was the same age as Emily, older than most of their peers, but she was the only one who had time off due to serious mental illness. On one of the pre-interview visits, the lead consultant in the department put a question to Emily: "Do you really think anyone would want to employ you, knowing that you have so few years to give back to the NHS as a consultant?"

He elaborated further by telling her that it would not be in the region's interests to spend their limited funds on training an older woman who was working part-time. It was disconcerting to hear a similar opinion from another male consultant at a different hospital and her confidence wavered.

But she defied them both by her success at interview, and she chose to start her first placement at Queen Alexandra Hospital in Portsmouth – the busiest A&E in the south of England. However, it had been enough to feel that she had to prove her worth and she capitulated to the pressure and agreed to shorten her training by working full-time.

## REASSESSMENT

One day following a busy shift, Emily walked through her front door to an assortment of shoes strewn over the hall carpet; the noise and laughter coming from the living room indicated that her teenage children had friends round. But that evening Emily longed for some peace and quiet; since starting the new job in November, she was finding it tough. When she came down with a nasty chest infection, it gave her the space to think, and she realised working full-time was too much. Fortunately, the postgraduate dean was sympathetic and facilitated her return to the flexible training scheme. Working part-time again would lead to a corresponding increase in the length of her postgraduate training. But Emily heeded the repeated warnings from her psychiatrists that she still faced a high risk of relapse, and she would do anything to avoid that; her health must be a priority.

## BOOK

Emily met a GP activist, who was a tremendous advocate for doctors suffering with mental health problems, and through him, Emily's story came to the attention of Radcliffe Publishing. It was still a surprise when she was approached with a publishing offer before she had decided to write a book. But this seemed like serendipity and despite the new job, Emily rose to the challenge. With a year to complete her memoir, Emily lay awake wondering how she was going to validate her recollections when she was also going to disclose that she had memory loss from ECT.

Fortunately, Emily had regularly kept a diary during the final eighteen months of the depression and had also written other pieces intermittently during those terrible years. She requested access to her medical records and planned to interview key members of staff. Undoubtedly it was going to be a challenge to remain authentic; to get the balance right between the reality of the mistreatment and bullying she had suffered during her hospital admissions, whilst simultaneously commending psychiatry for their valiant efforts in trying to keep her safe and make her better.

The DOP granted Emily access to her psychiatric records but only if they were viewed in the presence of her consultant; ostensibly so that he would be available to answer any questions.

It was arranged that Emily would peruse her notes during one of Dr Smith's outpatient clinics. It was a great comfort to have Peter with her when even the familiar NHS smell in that particular area of the hospital, triggered unpleasant feelings. Thankfully she did not have to endure the waiting room for long until Dr Smith ushered them into a room next door to his clinic. What greeted them was a tower of overflowing folders – six volumes of medical notes in all. Dr Smith left them to it, with the assurance that he would check back shortly. It felt odd to pick up the first folder. This was all about her and she had to face up to what others had written about what she was feeling and how she behaved, all from someone else's point of view. Peter and Emily sat themselves down and Emily turned the pages, wondering how she was going to take notes of what seemed relevant for her book when there was so much material. It was going to be impossible, and Peter suggested they return another time with a camera, ready to photo key pages which Emily could then refer to at her leisure. It was alarming to find one complete volume in the series was missing. Before they left, they managed to have a further chat with Dr Smith. He assured them that as a member of Southampton Hospital's staff, her notes were always kept in a locked filing cabinet. By their third visit Emily was increasingly apprehensive when it still hadn't been located.

Every time they came for a foray into her medical record, it became increasingly painful as more of Emily's experience emerged, written purely from the perspective of the medical or nursing staff. When she came across an entry suggesting that she was giving blades out to other patients for them to self-harm, she wanted to shout at the author, "That isn't true! How could you say such a thing?" It deeply offended her sense of morality. Another entry disputed her claims that she had been vomiting when she had a sick bug during one of the admissions. She remembered the way they had treated her and wished that the nurse who took the sick bowls away had made a record of her actions. Emily felt violated; her personal integrity had been so devalued.

Memories of hopelessness, lying curled up in a ball surrounded by horrible, brown, flowery curtains, wishing she would die, flooded to the surface. The knot in her stomach tightened every time she came across derogatory comments written in her notes. The lawyer who warned her off trying to sue the hospital was right. How could she possibly defend herself? Feeling very unsettled, Emily also worried that if she showed how much it was upsetting her, Peter or Dr Smith might suggest she abandon the writing.

## TRIGGERED

Sadly, Emily kept her feelings to herself, cutting Peter out and depriving herself of his much-needed support. She resolved to get the book finished as quickly as possible then at least she need not think about it any further. On the final information gathering session, Emily was on her own. Dr Smith made his usual enquiries about her health and this time Emily admitted that she wasn't sleeping well. He responded with alarm and though she was quick to reassure him that she wasn't feeling low or depressed and was still enjoying life, his furrowed brow betrayed his concern.

Emily knew the triggering of memories was affecting her alongside the job which was constantly tiring and stressful. But Dr Smith was not satisfied, and he explained to her that even if she wasn't feeling low right now, it was likely that she was on the brink of sliding back into depression. He described it as similar to having a migraine without the headache and advised that she start antidepressants immediately to 'nip it in the bud'. Emily hadn't heard of such a thing, but Dr Smith's anxiety was contagious and reluctantly Emily deferred to his expert knowledge. When he advised restarting venlafaxine, Emily said no. As a compromise, she agreed to take a drug she hadn't had before – trazodone. Dr Smith assured her that she would not suffer sexual side effects and it would also help with sleep. He wrote out a prescription and arranged for an official outpatient review.

Emily left, having just reacquired the status of psychiatric patient, while simultaneously writing a book about her spectacular recovery. She felt a complete and utter fraud.

Having capitulated, Emily attended the review appointment. Dr Smith was always meticulous, asking a battery of specific questions about sleep, appetite, weight, sex, concentration and mood, before he relaxed into general questions about work and enquiries on how the book was coming along. He always asked Emily about adverse effects from the trazodone and noted Emily's dry mouth on several occasions. Although she definitely slept better thanks to the sedating properties of trazodone, it also became a struggle to get up in the mornings. But now Dr Smith was able to reassure her that it was just a blip and that a potential recurrence of depression had successfully been averted.

## DISAPPOINTMENT

It felt like a weight had been lifted when Emily submitted the manuscript to the publisher, well before the deadline and more settled in her role at work, life had found a new and happy normal. Peter and Emily planned a party to celebrate their twenty-fifth wedding anniversary followed by a holiday with the family.

All seemed good until one day Peter came home in shock. He had gone to work as usual where he wrote specialist banking software. Without warning, strangers had walked into the office and announced they were the new management. Everyone was ordered to stop work. In order to qualify for the minimum redundancy payment required by law, Peter had to remain at his desk for another month but with nothing to do other than trawl the internet looking for jobs. It was soul-destroying. It also felt devastating as their future plans slipped away like sand through their fingers. Spending had to be reined in immediately and the holiday cancelled. Peter and Emily were dependent on both salaries, but Emily felt she couldn't risk becoming full-time again after the recent near miss.

Over the last few years, Peter's work had become extremely specialised; despite a degree and two decades of experience, he was pessimistic about his prospects of getting another job locally. The job market for computer programming had evolved and Peter lacked the academic credentials which most applications now demanded. It was frustrating when people tried to be helpful, suggesting job openings which were entirely unsuitable. It reminded Emily of the way non-medics couldn't fathom why a doctor working in one field of medicine found it so difficult to transfer to another speciality.

The redundancy pay only covered three months of Peter's salary and it was running out fast. Peter and Emily tried to remain cheerful and optimistic but concluded that now Steve was at university, Natalie was a student at Central school of Ballet in London and Harry was about to start sixth-form college, their best chance would be to make a fresh start. They decided to sell the house and move to a more affordable area.

## FRESH START

Emily thought it would certainly be a relief to get away from the constant reminders of the nightmare years in Southampton. But any move would be limited to an area which would accept a transfer of her A&E postgraduate training scheme. As they looked at the different options, Peter and Emily found themselves considering Scotland.

In September 2005, Emily had her annual follow-up appointment in Dundee for Professor Scott's continuing research. Peter and Emily decided to use the opportunity for a much-needed break. They found a wonderful bed and breakfast in Angus and every day that they were there, a rainbow appeared. It seemed like a sign that they were on the right track.

\* \* \*

*Perhaps it's not surprising that everyone was so anxious about Emily's mental health at this stage, but it seems possible that Emily's valid emotional responses to life's problems were misconstrued as relapse. Would you feel confident to question the advice you are given or discuss the decision to restart psychiatric drugs with your doctor? It is important that the risks as well as the benefits of any drug are discussed alongside the potential for serious and protracted withdrawal syndromes in advance of any decision to proceed.*

# CHAPTER 20

# Move to Scotland

The regions where Peter could look for work had to correspond with the areas where Emily could apply for an inter-deanery transfer of her A&E training. The stress was ratcheting up and despite taking trazodone, she felt anxious and unhappy. Just sitting on the orange padded chairs in the outpatient waiting room triggered her so much that Dr Smith scheduled further appointments in his office. He also referred her back to CBT, but to a different therapist who he assured Emily was both highly skilled and very experienced. These appointments were in the same building as the DOP wards and Emily felt caught between a rock and a hard place as feelings of panic rose in her chest before each visit. The therapist's remit did not include looking at the past or her coping mechanisms, instead he taught her mindfulness and meditation, while encouraging her to focus on the present.

## JOB-SEEKING

Radcliffe, Emily's publisher, planned the press release for *Life After Darkness* in the new year of 2006. Soon Emily's story of recovery would be in the public arena. Every time she had an appointment at the DOP, Emily kept her head down, avoiding eye contact, scared of being recognised. She chastised herself for succumbing to a relapse of depression and was greatly worried that it might reduce her chances of getting a successful inter-deanery transfer.

At last Peter had news of a job interview. Emily had already been in contact with the local deanery in north-east Scotland and she was told that economic migration was not an acceptable reason for an inter-deanery transfer. However, if her husband had already moved to the area, they might reconsider. The financial situation was rapidly becoming untenable, and even though Emily would rather continue her A&E training, she was also looking for any job she could apply for in the area. A staff-grade post in psychiatry in Aberdeen was advertised and stated that they were looking for a fresh approach to patient care and on-the-job training would be provided. Although Emily had not worked in psychiatry as a doctor, she applied on the basis that it had been her special interest in A&E; nonetheless she was surprised when she was short-listed and invited for interview.

But just as Peter was offered a job in the IT department at Aberdeen Royal Infirmary, Emily was happy to see a vacancy for an A&E registrar advertised at the same hospital. Emily was full of hope when she sent her CV to the deanery, along with a full and frank disclosure about her seven-year 'career break'.

When she came home after a late shift, she eagerly checked her emails for a response. Her blood ran cold as she read a reply stating that there were no vacancies for A&E registrars in Aberdeen and that there would not be any for the foreseeable future.

It seemed incomprehensible after she had clearly seen a vacancy advertised and Emily was tired and bitterly disappointed. She had heard many stories of discrimination against doctors with mental health problems and she made the mistake of composing an immediate reply. She asked whether the deanery had denied her the opportunity of applying for the advertised vacancy because she had disclosed a history of depression. And then she pressed send.

When she woke a few hours later, another email from the deanery was waiting in her inbox. It stated that they would not engage in any further communication with her. Emily was absolutely devastated. Clearly after the faux pas she had made, an inter-deanery transfer was now out of the question, and she had just ruined her chances of continuing her career in Emergency Medicine (A&E).

Panic-stricken, Emily immediately contacted her regional postgraduate dean and explained what had happened, and how she wanted to apologise for even considering the possibility that they would discriminate against her on the grounds of her psychiatric history. It was such a relief when her dean's intervention resulted in a direct invitation for Emily to visit the A&E department at the Aberdeen Royal Infirmary. They did indeed have a vacancy.

On paper, it seemed like a great place to work and despite the bad start, Emily hoped this visit would prove to be an opportunity to repair the damage and continue her postgraduate training. At the visit, Emily was shown around the A&E department and then ushered to a manager's office to talk about her future. He asked her why she still needed to work part-time since she no longer had young children. Emily answered honestly and explained that she had struggled when she had worked full-time (forty hours a week) at the start of her registrar post.

The manager's expression was less than friendly as he informed her that in Aberdeen full-time doctors worked fifty-six hours a week; he took out his calculator and told her that to work seventy per cent of full-time on the flexible training scheme, would equate to thirty-nine hours a week. Emily's salary would remain the same despite increasing her hours from twenty-eight to thirty-nine hours a week. He went on to say that she would not be allowed to disrupt the rota and she would be expected to work seven consecutive night shifts just like the full-time registrars. The bad news continued as he explained that all the registrars were also required to spend a minimum of one year, resident in the hospital in Inverness. He held up his hand when Emily started to object. There would be no concessions, none of it was up for negotiation.

Emily left his office reeling from shock. Her stomach churned, her mouth was dry, and her heart was racing. To end her visit, she was introduced to a doctor who would be one of her fellow A&E registrars. Alone in the coffee room, the registrar asked Emily whether she was accustomed to swearing. He elaborated further as he explained how this same manager made a habit of pushing newcomers to the edge, "until you tell him to f**k off publicly. You won't have to mind it," he said, "he picks on all new registrars. Don't take it personally. After that he'll leave you alone."

## CAREER CHANGE

Peter drove Emily to the airport to catch her return flight to Southampton, and she stared at the countryside in silence. Perhaps the increased hours would be tolerable, if it hadn't been for the warning that she was about to be bullied. As they entered a section of the winding road with evergreen forest on either side, suddenly Emily felt overwhelmed. She had already blotted her copybook with the deanery and there was nowhere to turn. "Stop the car!" she cried out.

Peter pulled into a siding and Emily burst into tears as she related all that had happened during the visit to A&E. It felt like clutching at straws, when trembling, she found the number for the secretary at the Royal Cornhill Hospital and asked if there was any chance that she could attend the interview for the staff-grade post in psychiatry, which she had previously declined. The secretary said she would make enquiries and let her know. They postponed her return flight and found a small hotel for the night. It seemed like serendipity that the interview was due to take place the following day.

The psychiatry consultants seemed so friendly in such contrast to her experience the day before. Emily confidently asserted that she could cope with working on a psychiatric ward, despite her experience as a patient. The job would be regular daytime hours, no nights, or weekends. The consultants assured her that they would train her up and she would not be expected to take charge of the ward and supervise the junior doctors until she was ready. Within the space of twenty-four hours, Emily had made a mind-boggling career change without consulting her usual confidantes, yet it felt such a relief.

Back at work, Emily put a positive spin on her sudden change in career direction as she handed in her resignation. Internally she felt torn in two; she weighed the regret over leaving Emergency Medicine against the alternative of working full-time hours, on part-time pay, while being supervised by a bully.

She felt really stupid after all the efforts her deanery had made to secure the inter-deanery transfer and ashamed of how successfully the manager had intimidated her. But she didn't think she would cope with being separated from Peter for over a year either. Emily buried her conflicting emotions, determined to press on, also mindful that showing distress might be interpreted as a sign of relapse and further jeopardise her future.

## FAMILY

Rachel was now married and living in London. Steve, their oldest son, was at university but living at home. Natalie was still a student at the Central School of Ballet in London, and Harry, aged seventeen, had already started sixth-form college. He was adamant that he did not want to move to Scotland. Steve and Harry wanted to live together in Southampton, which left Peter and Emily to console themselves that at least they would all meet up during the holidays.

Friends said their goodbyes when Peter left to start his job in Aberdeen, while Emily stayed behind in Southampton to work her three months' notice. It was stressful on her own and she constantly worried about leaving the boys in January, wondering how they would cope with laundry, cooking, and general housekeeping. Emily tried to gen up on psychiatry, as well as pack up the house; she paid little attention to the impending publication of her book.

Peter flew down to Southampton for their last family Christmas in the home where they had lived for the previous sixteen years. He had rented a two-bedroom flat in Torphins, a village outside Aberdeen, and assured Emily that the commute to work each day was beautiful, a drive through stunning countryside. Peter's return to Scotland in the new year coincided with the press release for *Life After Darkness*. But they weren't expecting much interest from the media.

## PRESS ATTENTION

It took Emily by surprise when the local Portsmouth paper asked if they could photograph her at Queen Alexandra Hospital where she worked. The *Southampton Echo* also requested a photo. It caused quite a stir when patients started arriving at A&E asking specifically if they could be seen by "Dr Wield, who had been in the paper". On her last day at work Emily felt something of a celebrity; it was surreal when suddenly her colleagues were interested in how she had survived severe mental illness.

The orders for *Life After Darkness* came in thick and fast and Emily was being asked to sign copies, while trying to say her goodbyes and finish the packing. Further requests for photos and interviews arose from the national press, which meant that those she accepted would have to be conducted from her new home in Scotland.

## RELOCATION

Early on the morning of Emily's departure, the boys helped her pack up the car. With the chili plant seat-belted to the front seat, she kissed them goodbye and drove away from their family home completely distraught, tears flowing down her cheeks. It wasn't the children who had flown the nest, it was their parents leaving them to fend for themselves. Emily cried for most of the ten-hour drive to Aberdeenshire and the grief felt like a kind of madness. It rained for the whole way which felt appropriate given her state of mourning.

It was dark by the time Emily arrived in Torphins and fell gratefully into Peter's arms. She had missed him so much while they were apart. But as she tried to unpack and settle in, her days were disrupted by photographers keen to find suitable places to conduct each unique photo shoot. The residents were bemused while a photographer equipped with all their paraphernalia took Emily around the village looking for the perfect place to take her photograph. Emily had no idea how to handle the publicity, she just wanted to get it over and done with before she started the new job. While she felt grateful for such positive press and the encouraging correspondence from strangers, she also felt very isolated. She missed the children, her friends and family. She knew nobody locally, apart from Peter; there was no one to fill the void or give her the support she longed for. With the media spotlight on her, Emily felt duty-bound to hide any distress. She felt she had no right to disillusion those who might find new hope as a result of her story of recovery.

## CORNHILL

The Royal Cornhill Hospital was a labyrinth of buildings joined by prefabricated walkways. There was a very distinctive smell as Emily walked into the large reception area. The tired-looking carpet, and an odd assortment of framed artwork on the walls contributed to a general aura of fatigue and neglect. Emily was immediately struck with how quiet it seemed in comparison to the hustle and bustle of an A&E department. She found herself trying to guess who's who, as she followed the directions to the ward where she would be based. Perhaps those walking faster or more purposefully were staff, confirmed only if she caught sight of a name badge. Maybe others who seemed in no hurry at all, could be her patients.

Emily's job was to provide clinical oversight of all the patients on one of the adult wards. They came from five different catchment areas in the region, each managed by individual consultant psychiatrists who oversaw their care. The first week was designated as orientation and Emily was given the opportunity to accompany some of the consultants to their outpatient clinics.

It was interesting to visit the north-east coast of Scotland, which was once home to thriving fishing communities. Restrictions imposed to conserve the fish stock in the North Sea had decimated the fishing industry, so many of the towns looked bleak with most shops and businesses boarded up. There was considerable disparity in socio-economic circumstances between these communities, compared to others who made a living from oil – big business in the city of Aberdeen itself.

Emily tried to absorb as much information as she could about the region, the local culture and of course, the practice of psychiatry. It took time to become attuned to the strong Aberdeenshire accents and some people spoke a local dialect called Doric. Emily found it difficult to understand both patients and staff alike. The consultants gave her books which they thought might enhance her knowledge of psychiatry, as well as copies of both the DSM (Diagnostic and Statistical Manual) and the ICD-10 (International Classification of Diseases). She was instructed to familiarise herself with the contents of the latter, as she would need to use the coding.

As a staff-grade doctor, Emily wasn't eligible for any formal training, but she was told she was welcome to attend any of the teaching sessions for junior doctors, which they could attend with protected time. For Emily, the stipulation was that her ward work must take priority and if asked, she must respond immediately to any urgent matters that needed attending to. A small room off the ward full of discarded bits of furniture was hastily appropriated as Emily's office, with promises that they would find what was needed to make it fit for purpose. It felt strange to be given a bunch of keys, granting access to the ward and other areas where patients were either locked in or kept out. The tables were turned and Emily had become one of the dreaded gaolers.

## HINDSIGHT

The sobering truth was that Emily's career had been thrown off course after an impulsive decision following a meeting with an intimidating manager. She had moved seven hundred miles away from friends and family whilst simultaneously becoming a focus of media attention. Then she started work in an environment likely to trigger memories of her recent experiences as a psychiatric patient. The problems of the past had never been dealt with, Emily's survival strategies from childhood were still very much in play. She had been started on antidepressants when her responses to the situation were very understandable. Now she had moved, Emily was supposed to be prioritising her health. Perhaps what followed should not have been any great surprise.

* * *

*Bullying should never be acceptable in the workplace. Corporations and institutions need to take their responsibilities seriously and tackle the culture which allows it to continue. Do you work in a psychologically safe environment? Are you able to identify significant stressors in your life? Have you found yourself dismissing factors which might have a bearing on your health and well-being?*

# CHAPTER 21

# Trouble brewing

One of the first questions Emily asked when she started her new job was where the resuscitation trolley was kept. The answer was alarming; when she was shown a plastic box containing a first aid kit and a couple of inhalers. When she shared her concerns about the lack of emergency equipment, she was reminded that she was employed as a psychiatrist, not as an A&E doctor and that her priority was to learn how to treat psychiatric conditions.

## WARD PSYCHIATRIST

As the days became weeks, Emily adjusted to the slower pace of work in her new job. Every week, each of the five consultants had a scheduled meeting known as a 'ward round', during which each of their patients would have their progress reviewed and their treatment planned for the coming week. Emily was expected to be present for every one of these five weekly meetings, each of which lasted several hours. In addition, representatives from the nursing staff, psychologists, psychotherapists, occupational therapists, and junior doctors associated with the consultant's team who contributed to their patients' care were also expected to be present.

The most recently admitted patients were discussed first to give sufficient time for deliberation over their diagnosis and subsequent drug treatment. Every patient review concluded with consideration of discharge readiness or if detained, plans for periods of leave outside the hospital, as well as medication changes. It was a team decision, but the consultant had the final say.

Emily was bewildered; it all seemed so precarious when the diagnosis was simply a matter of opinion. There were no tests or investigations to prove a psychiatric diagnosis, yet in the ward round, a patient's whole future could be determined by snippets of information and reports about what they had said or the way they behaved. Sometimes discussions became quite heated when opinions differed, whilst at other times a patient was given a diagnosis with alacrity. Equally puzzling was the way a prior psychiatric diagnosis was discarded if the current psychiatrist disagreed with it. Often at some point during the ward round, the unwitting patient was brought into the room and briefly questioned, their answers used to verify the prevailing theory. What alarmed Emily most, was the way a patient could suddenly be deemed to have a diagnosis of personality disorder, which seemed detrimental to their future care and would follow them for the rest of their life.

## SCEPTICISM

Emily also found her head spinning by the seemingly arbitrary decisions by which drugs were prescribed; very little logic seemed to govern their choices. Often the diagnosis seemed irrelevant, as patients were equally likely to be prescribed an antipsychotic as an antidepressant. The junior doctors were a great help because they were very familiar with the five consultants' prescribing habits.

Tranquillisers such as lorazepam were written up as a matter of routine, to avoid 'fuss', just in case the patient became agitated. Emily tried to suspend her disbelief as she found her faith in psychiatry beginning to crumble. As the least experienced member of the team, she was in no position to challenge accepted practice.

She rationalised that what she needed was more knowledge and more understanding. She was determined to get to grips with it all and started her education with the books on psychopathology and prescribing recommended by the consultants.

Meanwhile, Emily didn't find it easy to sign the drug charts having had first-hand experience of the awful adverse effects. But she had to believe the patients would benefit, knowing it was unusual for patients not to improve with treatment.

One thing she could do straight away was get to know every one of her patients on the ward and give them regular time to talk so she could advocate for their needs. Without fail, the patients appreciated her efforts, but it was disappointing how difficult it was to achieve her goal, given the busy schedule of meetings.

## PERSONALITY DISORDERS

When one of Emily's patients was readmitted with recurrent symptoms of severe depression and failed to improve despite several different combinations of antidepressants, it felt rather too familiar. During the weekly ward round, the patient's consultant mooted the idea of referring them to Cornhill's specialist in mood disorders, which led to a discussion on their diagnosis. Emily was gobsmacked as the staff vacillated over the option of making further efforts to treat depression or re-diagnose them with borderline personality disorder, in which case they would be discharged – 'not amenable to treatment'. Later the same day, the morning's debate was reignited by the staff as they sat in the large communal office, the central hub on the ward. One nurse was convinced that the patient had a personality disorder and backed it up by saying, "I saw them laughing on the phone," as if it was proof that the patient was malingering.

Tears filled Emily's eyes; she couldn't bear it any longer and fled to the privacy of her own office where she could get a grip on her emotions. Was this really the way patients were cared for in psychiatry? Very likely she had been the subject of similar machinations at the DOP.

Emily returned to the ward office and wrote her own entry in the patient record, referencing the patient's life before the onset of symptoms, a stable marriage, long-lasting friendships, and their work history. She wrote that there was no evidence of a personality disorder, and that the patient urgently needed an assessment by the consultant specialising in mood disorders.

I will write a caveat here. I do not believe that *any* patient, whatever their diagnosis should be treated badly or written off as a hopeless case without expectation of recovery. The label of personality disorder is exceptionally stigmatising and still has the propensity to prejudice patient care. Even though attitudes may have improved, the diagnosis of a personality disorder is one that sticks like glue and negatively biases the opinions of healthcare providers against the patient.

## SECOND THOUGHTS

Following Emily's psychosurgery in 2001, Professor Scott scheduled regular reviews and he also gave her an open invitation to update him by phone or email. When Emily attended appointments, they often spoke about stigma and the need to treat patients with compassion, kindness, and respect. Emily was disappointed that Professor Scott could not provide all of her psychiatric care, now they lived in Scotland.

The GP referred Emily to Dr Black who was the psychiatrist for her catchment area. He also worked at Cornhill and arranged to see her in one of her lunch breaks. Dr Black was pragmatic. He wasn't particularly concerned when Emily told him she was struggling and advised she continue trazodone at the same dose, but he did refer her for more CBT.

The CBT therapist didn't think there was anything further to be gained since she had had a course of CBT before she left Southampton. But work wasn't getting any easier and Emily was not happy with life. She emailed the only person she thought would understand, Professor Scott, saying she felt isolated and upset because she thought she was witnessing bad practice in her new role as a staff-grade psychiatrist.

Not knowing what else to do, Emily made an appointment to see Dr Max at Occupational Health. Dr Max told Emily he thought she should never have taken the psychiatry post in the first place and suggested she resign. Emily was mortified. How could she leave while they depended on her salary?

She wondered if there might be a way of resurrecting her career in Emergency Medicine, even if it meant returning to a more junior level and so she requested another meeting with the intimidating manager. What a mistake that was – it seems Emily hadn't clocked the seriousness of her offence. She had committed the medical equivalent of unforgivable sin by turning down the registrar job when she was offered the inter-deanery transfer. He laughed in her face and made derogatory comments about her mental health before he swore that he would make sure she never worked in any A&E in the region. She left the meeting outraged and decided to report him. It turned into a prolonged investigation, which added considerably to an already pressurised situation.

Every alternative that Emily explored, led to a dead end and she felt trapped in her current job. All she could do was resort to her usual coping mechanisms. She worked as hard as she could and tried to suppress her feelings.

## SCOTTISH LIFE

By May 2006, the house was sold, Peter and Emily returned to Southampton just to pack up and help move the boys to the place they would be renting. It was too late to turn back now and Emily tried to convince herself that she would be content living in their new house in Banchory for the rest of their lives. The living room was a good size with a south-facing window that overlooked a lawn and a circular flower bed at the front of the house. The two silver birches on either side were in leaf. It appeared peaceful and was certainly much quieter than living on the main road in Southampton.

They joined the local church where the congregation were welcoming and friendly. They met couples of similar ages, most of whom had raised their families in Banchory. During their annual leave, Peter and Emily made trips back to England, visiting the family they missed so much. Deep down, Emily knew it was unrealistic to expect their children to join them in this remote part of Scotland, however beautiful it was. But she clung to the hope that opportunities in Edinburgh or Glasgow might draw them a little closer. She also continued to hope that somehow, she would adjust to her new career as a psychiatrist.

## RELAPSE

The media flurry around *Life After Darkness* had been short-lived, but the patients and staff were intrigued when Emily was invited to appear on the Lorraine Kelly breakfast show. Emily felt a fraud knowing that currently her life was hardly one of happiness and contentment.

In October, Peter's mother came to stay for a week which Emily found a welcome distraction. But as soon as she left, Emily's bravado collapsed, and her GP signed her off sick with depression. Left with little to occupy her time, Emily analysed in detail how she had come to orchestrate this terrible mess. The slippery slope of self-doubt and self-blame set the downward spiral in motion.

Perhaps Emily's reactions were a valid response to her difficulties. Perhaps she could have made better choices. Perhaps it was made worse by a combination of bad luck and some extraordinarily unhelpful people. I wonder if it would have been any different if she was not programmed to expect a full-blown recurrence of depression.

I am sure the warnings from psychiatrists were well-intended – to make sure she received immediate, relevant treatment, but it backfired. Emily was scared of her feelings, which became worse once she went on sick leave. It rapidly escalated out of control, and unable to cope, Emily returned to the GP and told him she felt suicidal.

It was Dr Black who arranged for her admission to Carseview Centre in Dundee, back under the care of Professor Scott. This at least brought a modicum of relief, knowing that Professor Scott was someone who knew her, someone who Emily could trust. Peter, on the contrary, was not at all reassured. He couldn't understand how this could happen when God had supposedly healed her. Emily, on the other hand, thought God was not to blame when it was so obviously her fault.

The journey to Dundee was two hours long, crossing over a particularly high range of hills on winding roads with spectacular views of the heather-covered slopes. Emily called each of the children in turn and tried to make light of the situation. She completely failed to anticipate how infuriating her attempts at reassurance would be. Of course, another hospital admission was a big deal. They wanted to know why she hadn't been more open about the way she had been feeling.

By the time they arrived at the Carseview Centre, Emily was overwhelmed with regret and once admitted to the ward, there was plenty more time to contemplate her transgressions. She had let Peter and the children down. She had let Professor Scott's neurosurgical research down. As their 'star patient', she had exemplified the success of special interventions like brain surgery which could save other patients from their treatment-resistant depression. A whirlpool of shame sucked Emily under, and she genuinely wished she was dead.

Carseview was purpose built as a psychiatric unit shortly before Emily's admission for the surgery in 2001. The ward was mixed sex and most of the patients slept in single rooms. But Emily was admitted on a Friday evening and the only bed available was a shared room with another patient. Her roommate lost no time in telling Emily why she needed to have the radio on all night. When Professor Scott popped his head round the door before leaving for the weekend, he found Emily curled up on the bed in a foetal position, utterly miserable, not even prepared to raise her eyes to greet him. There was nothing to say, she had been given a second chance in 2001 and now had completely blown it.

## UNRESOLVED PROBLEMS

Whatever else had happened, the truth was that Emily's past problems had never been resolved. Her coping mechanisms were still as dysfunctional as ever, added to which was the more recent trauma from her seven years as a psychiatric patient. Emily stayed in bed all weekend and tried to block out the world. She refused to eat and drink. She couldn't sleep, intensely irritated by the other patient's radio.

On Monday, Professor Scott returned and told her she was extremely unwell with a serious relapse and must restart venlafaxine immediately. But Emily didn't want venlafaxine because of the awful adverse effects. He also suggested ECT but she didn't want that either because it had caused memory problems. It was then that Professor Scott introduced her to Graham, a specialist nurse-therapist on his team. Graham was warm and empathic and spent some time with Emily persuading her to comply with the treatment Professor Scott recommended. He conveyed the message that given the severity of her relapse, surely it was only reasonable to start an effective antidepressant like venlafaxine. Stressed out and afraid, Emily couldn't engage in any critical thinking. Reluctantly she capitulated.

They moved her to a single room, but Emily's relief was short-lived; there was an undeniable smell of stale urine which persisted even after she insisted that they make attempts to clean the carpet. The venlafaxine made Emily feel nauseated and she had no desire to eat or drink. Graham warned her that if she didn't agree to ECT, it was more than likely that the decision would be taken out of her hands. With the covert threat of detention under the Scottish Mental Health Act, because that was the only legal way that ECT could be given against her will, Emily finally gave consent.

## COERCION

Not surprisingly, as a combination of both the adverse effects of antidepressants and her dehydration, Emily's mouth was very dry, and she had difficulty swallowing. The anaesthetist decided that she must have an endoscopy to rule out a serious problem like cancer before she had ECT. Graham took Emily for a walk around the hospital grounds and asked her if she was worried. Emily replied that she hoped it was cancer and she would die. The shame of her relapse seemed more than she could bear, and

Emily could not imagine any kind of future now the memoir was published, when she was guilty of such duplicity.

The endoscopy was normal. Professor Scott personally supervised the ECT with the electrodes only applied to one side of her head, to reduce the risk of memory loss. While under anaesthetic, they used the opportunity to rehydrate Emily with intravenous fluids, but she only abandoned her food refusal when Professor Scott threatened to start her on olanzapine. Emily decided she would rather eat on her own terms than end up with drug-induced obesity again.

As the dose of venlafaxine was increased, Emily felt intensely restless; she paced up and down the ward with an awful feeling, like an itch seated deep down in her muscles. She couldn't sit still, couldn't sleep and life seemed intolerable. Professor Scott reassured her that it would soon settle as she got used to the higher doses and added zopiclone to the mix. He was pleased she was no longer lying in bed all day. She was eating and drinking and he thought her mood had also improved.

\* \* \*

*It can be challenging to draw a line between persuasion and coercion when psychiatrists believe their patients are seriously mentally ill and treatment will make them better. Although this becomes a moot point for patients who are formally detained under mental health legislation when they are no longer free to refuse treatment. In health services, a holistic and non-judgemental approach including a 'what matters to you' conversation has been shown to be effective for both patients and staff. Have you ever been asked, 'what matters to you'?*

# CHAPTER 22

# Scottish Christmas

Emily wasn't formally detained as a patient, but how voluntary she was, is debatable. The minute she disclosed suicidal thoughts to her GP, hospital admission was inevitable. She was admitted to a locked ward and any attempts to leave would lead to an immediate assessment. She knew the drill. First, they would try and persuade her to stay 'voluntarily', then if she refused, she risked a formal detention under the Mental Health Act. The system is by nature powerful and blatantly coercive.

## HOME LEAVE

Towards the end of December, Professor Scott 'granted' Emily leave from hospital, to join the family who were coming up to Banchory for Christmas. She tried to enjoy the festivities and mask her feelings, but she was still dominated by guilt and shame and continued to berate herself for ruining their lives.

One cold, dark, and frosty afternoon, they were sat at the dinner table. Peter was engaged in a heated debate with Emily's parents and the children excused themselves. Emily felt stressed by the tension, and nobody noticed her slip out of the house. She must have seemed so selfish when they discovered she was missing. The family were so worried as they searched, and Emily was so blind to how triggered they were by her 'relapse'.

Nonetheless, it is hard to describe the overwhelming anguish she felt or explain the degree of torment which completely dominated her. Once again stuck in repetitive cycles of obsessional thoughts, Emily felt out of control for hours or days at a time. She was probably suffering with akathisia as a result of the increasing doses of venlafaxine.

It is not unusual for friends and loved ones to find it difficult to relate to or even imagine the intensity of such distress which in turn can lead to further misunderstandings between patients and their families. In this instance, Emily, the person at the centre of their concern, was so wrapped up in her distress that she became oblivious to the needs of her loving family.

Nobody, it seems, professionals or not, were aware that antidepressants had never helped Emily. If anything, these drugs increased her propensity to feel suicidal. As before, the prescribers gave the same message that she would soon feel better and when she didn't, Emily had every reason to feel incredibly frightened.

Despite the high dose of venlafaxine and having undergone a course of ECT, Emily failed to bounce back, and she was petrified that once again she would be stuck in 'treatment resistance'. The real Emily had disappeared from view, and she wondered if she was destined to be a psychiatric patient for the rest of her life.

The family all returned back to their lives in the south; Emily returned back to the psychiatric unit in Dundee. Without any explanation, Emily discovered that Professor Scott was no longer overseeing her care. She felt rejected, wondering what she had done wrong. Later, she found out that Professor Scott had withdrawn because he thought he was becoming too involved; but they could hardly tell Emily that, could they?

## TRAPPED

Meanwhile, Emily's circumstances hadn't changed. She was still trapped in the impossible conundrum of her own making. The antidepressants may have dumbed down her emotions, but that didn't solve her problems or equate to feeling better. She just felt numb and exceedingly disappointed by all her failures. As soon as her head hit the pillow each night, her mind came alive. Always a pro at rumination, she went over and over her deficiencies and intensely restless, sleep evaded her. To counteract this, the dose of her sedative antidepressant, trazodone, was increased to unlicensed high doses. Whatever symptom Emily reported, she was told it was a sign of just how ill she was, yet so much of what she experienced could just as easily have been attributed to the adverse effects of her medication.

There was nothing to do and Peter was prohibited from bringing Emily a portable TV because it was 'against hospital policy'. Despite her voluntary status, Emily wasn't allowed to leave the ward unless accompanied by a member of staff. She was going stir-crazy with far too much time to focus her attention on anything and everything that was bad about her life.

The minister from their Banchory church drove the four-hour round trip to visit her and some of the church members sent Emily cards and little gifts to cheer her up. She hardly knew some of the women who volunteered to help Peter out by coming to collect her, when she was allowed home for weekend visits. Emily was incredibly touched by the kindness and support from the church community.

## NEGLECTED

One night, Emily heard a fellow patient, we'll call Marjory, coughing more than usual. Marjory's room was just across the corridor and when she cried out, Emily went to check on her. Marjory was a heavy smoker, and Emily immediately recognised her laboured breathing was a sign she needed urgent medical attention and she summoned the nurses. But she couldn't relax when she heard one of the nurses saying, "Marjory, what are you doing wetting the bed? Do you expect us to clean up for you when you're perfectly capable of going to the toilet."

Thoroughly alert, Emily waited, hoping they had already called the doctor. When she realised no one was coming, she went back to Marjory's room and found she'd deteriorated further. This time Emily ran down the corridor and insisted the nurses get help immediately. It was such a relief when the paramedics collected Marjory to ferry her by ambulance, the short distance across the road to A&E at Ninewells Hospital. It was terrifying that qualified psychiatric nurses lacked the skills to recognise serious illness.

This was not the only cause for concern when it came to patients' physical welfare. When the cleaner left her trolley in the corridor and brought a bucket containing a toilet brush and several cloths hung over the side, into Emily's en-suite bathroom, she watched horrified. The cleaner used one of the cloths to clean the toilet seat, lift it up, wipe what was beneath it before using the same cloth to wipe the basin and taps. From then on, Emily watched her like a hawk. It happened every time and Emily found herself obsessionally recleaning, whenever the cleaner thwarted Emily's attempts to stop her from cleaning her room. Emily took her concerns to the ward manager. "It's not my business to interfere with the domestic staff," the manager said and advised Emily to bring it up at the patient discussion group. Collectively the patients sent an urgent communication to the hospital management asking for an immediate response. Management failed to reply or honour invitations to discuss the matter further. Nothing changed.

## OVERDOSE

The system was so oppressive, and Emily heard other patients say they felt both ignored and disrespected. Plagued by adverse effects, Emily continued to worry about the future, and she felt overwhelmed by the hopelessness of her situation. One cold, February day she managed to slip out of the ward unnoticed. Without any clear idea of where she was going, she took the first bus that stopped on the road outside. It was headed away from Dundee, and she got off when it reached a small town, where she spotted a supermarket. Emily went round the tills twice buying pain relief and a bottle of Coke. After she had taken all of them as an overdose, she realised there was nowhere else to go. Without cards and very little cash, she decided she might as well return to die in the warmth of the ward.

Her outing had gone unnoticed. But now she was back, Emily felt ambivalent about her impulsive and reckless overdose and decided to confess about what she'd done. In response, two nurses came to search her room and when they found nothing amongst her belongings and no evidence of empty packaging, they clearly didn't believe her.

Emily was filled with remorse, thinking how ironic it was that she had actually managed to take a decent overdose and now she would die because the hospital was so incompetent.

Then all of a sudden, a nurse came and moved Emily to a room nearer the nurses' station and an HCA (healthcare assistant) was posted outside her door. A junior doctor came in to take blood, but since no one had asked her any of the details, Emily knew from her medical training that the results would be inaccurate. The painkiller levels could only be interpreted if the sample was taken at least four hours after the overdose. She wrote letters to her family telling them she was sorry.

The ringing in Emily's ears became so loud that she could hardly hear anything, and she started vomiting. The doctor returned and assured her that her blood levels were fine. Emily didn't want to die, she just wanted it all to stop, and she made up her mind that if she survived, she must never, ever be so stupid again. She begged him to repeat the blood test and had to spell out step by step, why the first blood sample had been taken too soon.

Emily was very unwell by the time they transferred her to A&E. She was grateful that she received treatment but also very ashamed of what she had done. The following day when she was discharged back to Carseview, the overdose wasn't even mentioned. Nobody asked what had tipped her over the edge but instead, Emily had earned herself a stint on 'obs' (constant observation), not allowed to leave her room. Filled with angst and remorse, she apologised for causing so much trouble, but the nurse outside her door didn't pay any attention.

## OBSERVATION

While she remained on 'obs', the nurses rarely talked with her, though sometimes they talked about her. Most of the time, they just talked to each other and at night made little attempt to lower their voices. There was usually someone on constant obs, and quite often other patients would become so fed up with the noisy nurses that the night-time disturbance was made even worse by the loud confrontation that followed.

The only significant interaction Emily had with a nurse was when she would come into the room so they could directly observe her when she used the toilet or shower. It was humiliating. Thankfully after a few days, Emily was granted toilet privacy; that is until Hilda took a turn outside her door.

Hilda had a bad reputation amongst the patients. She

always sat on a towel because she thought the chairs used by patients were too dirty for her to sit on directly. While she sat outside Emily's room, Hilda complained loudly what a waste of time it was. But as soon as she spotted Emily going into her en-suite bathroom, she got up and followed her inside. Emily explained she needed privacy and asked Hilda to leave. Hilda refused. Emily assured her that she was safe, and she wouldn't harm herself. Still Hilda refused. Emily asked Hilda to fetch one of the trained nurses, but Hilda said no. When Emily tried to leave her room to find someone herself, Hilda barricaded the door and refused to let her out.

Suddenly Emily lost her cool. She was scared at being imprisoned in her room and started shouting and screaming just to get someone's attention. At last, one of the trained nurses arrived and only after Emily had calmed down was she able to tell Debs what had happened. Debs immediately gave Emily the privacy she needed to go to the toilet. Afterwards she defended Hilda's actions, explaining how hard she found it to 'take the risk'. Emily knew otherwise. The other patients had a nickname for Hilda with her dominating and cruel ways... But probably Hilda did Emily a favour because it gave her the determination to get out of the place before it drove her crazy.

Professor Scott resumed charge of Emily's care, and understood how hard it was for her to hold onto any kind words that were said, or remember any sort of validation of her distress. To counter this, he wrote in her diary, *You are not bad, you are seriously ill.*

\* \* \*

*What has your experience been? I hope that you are receiving a holistic and patient-centred approach to your care. It is important to be respected and to have your opinions listened to. Have you heard of advocacy services? (See appendix.)*

# CHAPTER 23

# The lecture

Perhaps it was a supreme irony that Emily received an invitation to speak to nursing students at the university of Southampton. She prepared notes for the lecture which Peter delivered on her behalf.

Yet much of what she wrote then remains relevant, even today:

\* \* \*

*"I have never been exuberantly extrovert but I was nonetheless outgoing. I enjoyed company, had good friends, loved going out but guess what? When I was feeling depressed, I was none of those things – I became intensely introverted and therefore unwittingly self-centred. I retreated into myself, avoided company and yet when faced with those I loved and cared for, would put on a 'good face'. The patient must be understood whatever the context of their lives and circumstances, both when they feel fine and when they feel symptomatic.*

*"Most hospitals in the UK are located in an urban*

environment; probably for ease of access but the truth is that they often lack space, and the facilities are inadequate. Very little attempt is made to improve the environment and make the best of what is present. The décor is often depressing in itself, dilapidated and the need for redecoration is low priority. Even though Carseview had not been open long, the carpets and chairs were smelly. When one of my fellow patients was incontinent on a chair, the covers weren't removed, and it wasn't taken out of circulation; we had to live with the consequences. Whereas I could hardly blame one of the staff for sitting on towels whenever they used the furniture, it still made me feel that us patients were less than; we weren't afforded such a privilege.

"Communal and individual bathrooms and toilets for psychiatric patients require the same hygiene standards that would be acceptable to members of staff. It is important that the ancillary staff in psychiatric hospitals are employed in the understanding that the needs of psychiatric patients are of equal importance to the needs of patients anywhere. When nursing staff are not interested in these concerns, they are letting patients down.

"Hospitals often lack adequate provision for patients to take exercise and/or they don't factor in that enough personnel are required to allow patients time outside. While the literature pushes the benefit of exercise in the prevention and treatment of mental health conditions, these very same patients are denied access to it. Does this make any sense?

"The food in hospital was appalling. It was cooked off-site, brought in as 'ready meals', which were then heated up in their plastic containers. Nothing was fresh, the quality of the meat was terrible; it seems the importance of a healthy diet was patently ignored for patients who might spend weeks or months in hospital.

"The noise at night was terrible. The nursing staff who were posted outside the doors of patients who were on twenty-four-hour observation ('suicide' watch), made little effort to keep their voices down. Sometimes I heard other patients lose their tempers with staff during the night and when a shouting match ensued, it made everything worse than ever. When I brought this up with the nurse in charge – she said, 'this was their daytime', so I should not expect night staff to keep quiet. The importance of sleep was not respected, and the only way insomnia was dealt with, was to prescribe medication.

"The way the body habituates to the effects of medication inevitably led to the need for increasing doses to get me to sleep. As a consequence, I would find myself unable to get up in the morning and feeling hungover during the following day.

"There were plenty of notices around the ward on how you could make a complaint – yet doing so did not change anything, other than earn you the label of a troublemaker or nuisance. Patients' rights were not seen as important and those of us who made an effort to get improvements made were not respected or taken seriously.

"I can't help wondering, would hospice patients be treated like this? Or patients on a cancer ward? Surely, we deserve equal standards of care to other patients. Furthermore, the inpatient psychiatric wards are described as being a therapeutic environment. What a joke.

"We had been given diagnoses and told that our illnesses were caused by such things as chemical imbalances in our brains. We might be 'mentally ill' but if mental health services really believed that the problem was in our physical brain, what was the logic that led to us being treated differently to other patients with other physical conditions?

"I am glad that the conditions under which I had the ECT have improved from a safety perspective. But ECT has never been proved to be reliable and effective, despite what the proponents claim. Furthermore, I was coerced into giving consent. When I first had ECT, I was like most patients, completely unaware of how damaging it is to memory. I lost important memories as a result of this treatment and now they are gone forever.

*"Patients were restrained on the ward quite frequently. Thankfully, I never had to go through that."*

## INADEQUATE AFTERCARE

*"Most completed suicides occur after recent discharge from hospital. Doesn't this speak volumes that hospital care does not make people better?"*

## THE BIGGEST BARRIER OF ALL – STAFF ATTITUDE

*"I have heard it said during the course of my work – 'it's not illness, only behaviour'! Staff in psychiatric units usually treated the patient with more compassion while they believed the patient was 'unwell' but the moment they believed that the patient had a modicum of control, then the way the patient responded or acted out, was labelled 'behaviour'. This led to the staff in turn responding either in a punitive way, showing displeasure and even using deterrents such as close observations as punishment or else the patient was simply ignored.*

*"I think that there should be more trained staff; those who are untrained may be excusably ignorant of mental illness and it increases their susceptibility to copying the bad attitudes displayed by some staff. I would not pretend that looking after psychiatric patients is an easy job and undoubtedly staff are subjected to abuse, probably more so than in any other branch of medicine. However, they still need to remain professional despite this. In good hospitals, the staff are all invited to a 'group' session, to discuss their feelings especially in relation to challenging patients.*

*"I know there are many fantastic untrained staff but even so, it should not be forgotten that they are untrained. Often it is these untrained healthcare assistants, who do the bulk of the caring roles, which place them in direct patient contact. It may be difficult for the trained staff to leave their paperwork and*

*therefore leave their office as often as they would like, but patients are not aware of why this is; when trained nurses aren't available, it may be perceived as neglect or rejection. Patients are savvy and easily get to know who the good staff are. This is a constant topic of conversation amongst themselves. On the ward there was a particular healthcare assistant who abused her position and was able to wield an unhealthy amount of influence even over the trained staff. She epitomised a judgemental and uncaring attitude. She ruled the roost at many of the mealtimes and was positively vile to certain patients. I couldn't understand why her colleagues put up with her. I was never quite sure whether staff like that went into the job already harbouring such attitudes or whether it was a manifestation of burn-out. It may be understandable that a bad decision is made when employing someone who is untrained, but surely it is inexcusable when it comes to trained staff.*

*"When I was last admitted, I thought it was supposed to be a hospital, not a correction centre. I hoped that none of these nurses went into their profession to punish patients. Nursing staff, medical staff and even untrained nursing or healthcare assistants need to refrain from being judgemental. That is not part of the job description.*

*"I always worried when I heard cynicism expressed over the caring attitudes showed by the seemingly naïve nursing or medical students. 'They'll soon learn!' says a more experienced member of staff, who clearly does not approve of their ability to be kind. Once a staff member's innate goodness and kindness is lost to cynicism, surely the work becomes less enjoyable and yes, the patients will notice, even if their fellow staff don't want to.*

*"The 'them and us' attitude continues to be pervasive within all medical services which when taken to extremes becomes: them (patients) equals inferior and undeserving, versus us the staff, equals superior and deserving. It can be particularly destructive on psychiatric wards. It promotes the belief that dealing with life's difficulties 'would never happen to me' and I suspect this may be*

one of the reasons that people leave the profession or hide their own difficulties. I want all staff everywhere to think about how they would like to be treated if they were feeling awful, whether sad, anxious, unhappy, isolated, or lonely.

"If only all our NHS hospitals could be like the Priory hospitals, notwithstanding the fact that such care costs money. I do believe that within the NHS, there is a myth that if psychiatric patients are too comfortable, then they will resist discharge home. Clearly if a patient prefers living in an institutional setting with consequent loss of independence, then that is another problem which psychiatry should be supremely placed to tackle. The priority for all staff caring for patients who are being treated within the psychiatric system must be to make sure that their patients are listened to, respected, and treated with dignity."

* * *

If you were going to give a similar lecture, how would you describe your own experiences?

# CHAPTER 24

# Banchory

Emily forged new friendships during the lifts home with women from the Banchory church and it helped pave the way for a successful discharge. The six-month admission had been a cogent reminder of just how awful it was to be a psychiatric patient and Emily felt extremely relieved to be home.

## NEW THERAPY

Undoubtedly it was challenging to distance herself from the role of 'vulnerable' psychiatric patient and become established in the local community as an independent, free-thinking and 'sane' individual. But as Emily's confidence grew, she felt more like her old self again. Admittedly she was hampered by severe daytime sedation and often didn't get out of bed until midday. The world never felt quite real, and she was aware how numb she felt. Professor Scott said it indicated that she was still very depressed.

Emily's diagnosis was changed to 'recurrent major depressive disorder' and Professor Scott counselled Emily to accept the inevitability of further relapses with a high risk of future hospitalisations. As before he opined that the relapse was 'endogenous' i.e. caused by a chemical imbalance and/or subtle structural abnormalities in her brain and only amenable to treatment with medication and ECT.

Professor Scott was clear that the priority was relapse prevention, and he was adamant that there was no benefit in revisiting Emily's past with psychotherapy or counselling.

Professor Scott recommended CBASP (Cognitive Behavioural Analysis System of Psychotherapy) to enhance Emily's coping skills as well as identify and avoid triggers. Despite the arduous nature of the four-hour round trip to Dundee every week, Emily looked forward to the sessions with Graham, the consultant nurse-therapist who she had already met on the ward. He was very empathic as a therapist, and optimistic as he tried to persuade Emily what a talented and worthwhile person she was.

On the drive home, Emily found plenty of time to reflect; she wrestled with his views, wondering how she could accept his concept of innate goodness, while as a Christian she had been taught to believe she was a sinner. But Graham's kindness did wonders for her self-esteem, and alongside Professor Scott's insistence that she had a 'biological' reason for her depression, it helped annihilate her continued suspicion that both the original years of depression and this subsequent relapse were somehow her fault.

Graham was tasked with co-creating a 'relapse signature' for Emily, to help identify early warning signs that she was becoming unwell again, and he assisted the writing of an advanced directive on how she would like to be treated during future hospital admissions. But every time Emily strayed into the realm of her childhood difficulties, Graham reminded her that she could only talk about current problems as talking about the past was off-limits.

## CLAN GATHERING

During the summer of 2007, Peter and Emily went with church friends to a Christian conference in St Andrews called the 'Clan Gathering'. One of the keynote speakers described his feeling of abandonment when he was sent away to boarding school at a young age. He went on to talk about his lack of a close and loving relationship with his father, and surmised that unwittingly he had projected his feelings about his dad onto 'God the Father'. This resulted in symptoms later in life which he termed 'an orphan heart', many of which sounded remarkably similar to Emily's symptoms of depression. Mark Stibbe was a powerful and charismatic speaker, and had written several Christian books. His message had a profound impact on Emily and again raised the possibility that her own troubled childhood could be responsible for some of her symptoms. Yet this Christian leader hadn't been treated as someone who was mentally ill. He saw it as a spiritual condition, and invited people to come to the front for healing prayer. Emily responded and even though nothing dramatic happened, she came away feeling uplifted. It was the first hint that others also suffered as a result of being sent away to boarding school.

At the next appointment, Professor Scott noticed a change. Emily put it down to the Clan Gathering experience but he put it down to the increased dose of venlafaxine.

Emily continued the weekly sessions with Graham and continued to comply with the medication. She was prescribed high doses of venlafaxine 600mg, trazodone 300mg (both unlicensed), as well as flupentixol and zolpidem. Professor Scott was insistent that this drug regime should continue at the same doses for the foreseeable future. He repeatedly told Emily that she would need to take antidepressants for life. Somewhere Emily heard the mantra, 'What gets you well, keeps you well'.

## DIFFERENT INTERPRETATIONS

The psychiatric paradigm invariably led to medicalisation of feelings which could be interpreted in a number of ways. For example, when Emily reported the feeling of numbness, it was reworded as *emotional blunting*. If she said she wasn't enjoying life, it was *anhedonia* and the persistent feeling that the world wasn't real, was *derealisation* and *depersonalisation*. Her tiredness and fatigue were again used as further proof that she was still depressed. It is curious that none of these symptoms were considered just as likely to be the adverse effects of the high doses of her psychiatric drugs.

It took a lot of courage to bring up the matter with Professor Scott of her unsatisfactory sex life. It felt profoundly uncomfortable to discuss her inability to orgasm, but Emily knew it was a direct effect of venlafaxine. While he did not disagree altogether, Professor Scott was quick to reassure her that as the depression improved, so would her libido. He argued that her depression had been so serious, that it was far better to be relatively well by taking venlafaxine than enjoy sex. In short, tolerating the adverse effects had to be worth it. Emily wondered whether he would say the same thing to a male patient complaining of drug-induced impotency, but she didn't dare voice her thoughts when she felt so indebted to Professor Scott and Graham. They had both shown a great deal of empathy, were consistently kind, compassionate, attentive and never judgemental, which in Emily's experience was most unusual.

She never suspected them of being specifically sexist towards her as a woman, but she knew only too well that medicine was culturally sexist, and psychiatry was perhaps the worst offender. After all, Viagra had been researched and funded to help men, but even talking about women's sexual problems was taboo.

## GRATITUDE

Emily always felt extremely grateful to Professor Scott and the team at AIS for their flexibility and the way they were so responsive to her needs. Other patients who had failed to respond to conventional psychiatric treatments also valued the AIS team. Jeannie was a patient Emily met during her admission who had also undergone brain surgery for intractable depression; a long-term friend, she also echoed Emily's admiration of Professor Scott and thought Graham was an extraordinary therapist. At a later date, they organised a patient group to nominate both Professor Scott and Graham for awards as outstanding professionals working in mental health services.

While Emily admired and trusted Professor Scott's judgement more than any of her previous psychiatrists, it probably made it harder to be assertive or independent over her treatment decisions. She was still under the impression that her relapse had been a disappointment for the research into neurosurgery as a treatment for mental disorder. In retrospect, Emily's desire to please and her perception that they accepted her *despite her failure,* increased her deference to their opinions. Perhaps Professor Scott and Graham were like father figures who plugged a hole in her life, left by a childhood devoid of affirmation and encouragement.

## MORE PLANS

Occupational Health recommended Emily's medical retirement from her job. Professor Scott supported this and advised that she should be subjected to as little stress as possible. He warned Emily that a return to work would put her at considerable risk of relapse. But Emily hadn't completely given up on herself and still held out the possibility that she might return to work in the NHS at a later date. It was a race to get the paperwork to the relevant authorities before the rules were due to change. They made it with less than twenty-four hours to spare.

Peter was reconsidering his future career and finding himself eligible for a student loan, applied for a degree course in London which combined his dual interests in theology and counselling, approved by the British Association for Counsellors and Psychotherapists (BACP).

Initially Emily wondered how she would cope with yet another move, but a return to England would bring them closer to the family they missed so much, and they were going to be grandparents. She had also begun to realise that she was becoming overly dependent on the Dundee team. Even though she would miss the regular sessions with Graham, it was a good opportunity to stand on her own two feet.

Professor Scott was pleased with Emily's progress and considered her 'stable' on the current drug regime. But given the poor prognosis of relapsing and remitting depression, he was insistent that she needed ongoing psychiatric care to monitor her condition. Emily hoped she would find another empathic psychiatrist who would take a personal interest in her case.

It would be the new GP who would have to initiate a referral to local services which left a period when Emily could fall through the cracks. Both Professor Scott and Graham offered to maintain contact by phone or email while Emily settled into her new life and encouraged her to monitor her mood and report any changes.

\* \* \*

*Do you identify with the downsides of feeling dependent on healthcare professionals who are supporting you? Have you found the right balance between continuity of care and your own autonomy? Many people feel betrayed or abandoned when there are changes in staff. Sometimes finding peer support may help.*

# PART 3

# Radical rethink

# CHAPTER 25

# Northwood

Peter and Emily rented a flat in Northwood, near to Peter's college. It was only just a few miles away from both of their daughters who lived in London and both of whom now had babies. Steve was also married and lived in Southampton. Harry, their youngest son, had surprised them all, when he chose to go to bible school in America, rather than take up his place at university. They all assumed he would return to England afterwards, but always an entrepreneur at heart, Harry thrived in the American culture. He was offered a job and never returned to live in the UK.

## TURBULENCE

Peter settled into college life while Emily unpacked and organised the flat. Initially she was buoyant with the move but felt alarmed when she started to feel a bit fed up. Graham had worked with her on a 'relapse signature' and a change in mood was potentially an ominous sign. When both the GP and the chemist questioned the high doses of venlafaxine and trazodone, Emily referred them back to Professor Scott who initiated the prescription. Once reassured that the unlicensed doses were truly his recommendation, they issued the drugs without further ado and Emily was referred to the local psychiatrist.

When the appointment eventually came through, Emily was disappointed. Dr Shy seemed to be the polar opposite to her team in Dundee. After a brief introduction during which he explained that the Trust had gone paperless, Dr Shy swivelled his chair round to type answers into his laptop which was on the desk behind him. He only turned back to face her occasionally while clarifying a detail.

When Emily received a copy of the clinic letter addressed to the GP, she was appalled by the number of factual errors. She asked Dr Shy to correct the mistakes, but it did not fill her with confidence. Emily wondered what she would do in the event of another relapse.

There was an emergency helpline number if she needed contact between appointments and one day, feeling particularly low, Emily gave it a try. An unenthusiastic voice read Dr Shy's erroneous notes back to her, without any hint of concern or validation of what she was feeling. Emily reached out to Professor Scott in desperation, and he confirmed her worst fears. He thought she was definitely becoming unwell again and arranged for the GP to increase the dose of flupentixol.

At least Dr Shy had made it clear that he was more than happy to defer to Professor Scott since he had no experience of patients like Emily who had had psychosurgery or were on such high doses of venlafaxine and trazadone. Perhaps it was fortuitous when a letter from Professor Scott went astray suggesting the addition of quetiapine to her cocktail of medication.

## PRIVATE COUNSELLOR

Relocation is a stressful life event and once again Emily was socially isolated with little to occupy her time. It wasn't helped by a visit from the benefits agency, to inform her of their overpayment error and how they now needed to recover the money.

None of the psychiatrists made any attempt to normalise Emily's feelings, but Dr Shy suggested she find herself a counsellor privately since she failed to meet the criteria for community support from psychiatric services.

Since Peter was now a student without an income, Emily was reticent to pay for a counsellor. However, Joe saw her at a concessionary rate. But he readily admitted that he didn't understand Emily's complex psychiatric history or her treatment. It was the first time that Emily had experienced any counselling/ psychotherapy outside NHS psychiatric care. She had become used to the partnership which existed between Graham and Professor Scott where they continuously exchanged information.

When Joe suggested that they explore her childhood past, she was worried. Graham had discouraged this on numerous occasions. Nevertheless, she cooperated when Joe presented her with a large sheet of paper and coloured pencils, to draw a timeline from birth to the present and illustrate major life events along the way. Despite the initial reluctance, Emily was struck by the number of significant events throughout her life. Joe suggested that they look at these in more detail, but Emily's anxiety over their financial situation got the better of her. She knew it would take some time and still conflicted by the Dundee team's advice, she terminated the sessions with Joe.

## SIDE EFFECTS

In an email to her friend, Jeannie, Emily wrote she had an *awful, unsettled feeling* like an *itch in my head but I don't know where to scratch*. She was surprised when Jeannie replied that she too experienced similar feelings. Neither of them knew that this unpleasant sensation was very likely attributable to the high doses of venlafaxine which they both took at the behest of their mutual psychiatric team in Dundee. Emily also continued to feel numb, and that the world was not quite real, but she also realised that the time of crisis had passed. She made new friends in the local community and began to enjoy the cosmopolitan life of outer London.

It had dawned on Emily a while back that it was the drugs that were causing her debilitating daytime fatigue, but she was also very bothered by the continued sexual side effects. She knew the latter had nothing to do with depression or low libido and proved it convincingly when she missed a few doses of venlafaxine. Armed with irrefutable evidence, she plucked up courage and rang Professor Scott. This time she was frank and told him she knew that venlafaxine prevented her from experiencing orgasm. His answer was the same as before. "Yes, it *may* be true but…" Professor Scott was quick to remind Emily of how ill she had been. He counselled that reducing the dose of venlafaxine was extremely risky, especially after her recent dip in mood.

But discussing her sex life was never an easy topic with anyone, let alone a male doctor and she let it pass. The suggestion that just being close to Peter was 'enough', always left Emily feeling frustrated and angry. Since many more women than men are prescribed antidepressants, she wondered how many of them were in the same boat.

## DISCONTENT

The chairs lined the walls in the dingy waiting room. It was pretty quiet as people avoided each other's gaze, keeping heads down, paying a lot of attention to their phones or turning pages of well-thumbed magazines. Suddenly a woman burst through the door and asked if anyone else was about to see Dr Shy.

Without waiting for a response, she announced, "He's bloody useless, zero bedside manner."

After her own appointment, Emily admitted she couldn't agree more and put in a request to see a different psychiatrist in future. She was assigned to his registrar for the next couple of appointments. But when the registrar moved on, Emily received a letter from Dr Shy inviting her to come and discuss the reasons she no longer wished to see him. When Emily declined his offer, she was told there was no other choice; allocation to a particular psychiatrist was done according to the catchment area where she lived.

Emily wrote to her MP and asked why patients had no choice over which psychiatrist they saw, while in every other branch of medicine, a patient could choose to change doctor if they wanted to. The MP was sympathetic and six months after he intervened, Emily finally received a response from the Trust saying they would find her an alternative psychiatrist. But they warned her, she would have to travel further to a different venue. The new psychiatrist was warm-hearted, empathic and about to go on maternity leave. Later, Emily put herself forward and was elected as a patient-governor to the Trust, determined that psychiatric patients should be served better.

## NEXT STEPS

Peter and Emily tried to sell their house in Scotland, but the financial crash of 2008 hit the housing market hard. The sale fell through and the income from letting the house in Banchory turned out to be much less than anticipated. Emily tried to stay positive while they repeatedly lowered the house price without securing a sale.

One of the neighbours introduced Emily to a senior A&E doctor who worked in nearby Watford. Emily wondered if she would ever work again after Professor Scott's advice, and with the consensus of opinion of her grim prognosis and likely relapse. She knew she had to be realistic and whatever happened she would first need to reduce doses of her drugs to lessen the daytime sedation.

Then suddenly everything changed. Their daughter urgently needed help with childcare and considering how much she owed her children, this seemed like a golden opportunity. Emily was delighted by this chance to look after her grandchild.

## ALARMING RESEARCH

Around the same time, Emily read a very worrying article in the *BMJ*. Research had demonstrated an increased mortality for those prescribed long-term antipsychotics and Emily had been taking flupentixol for several years already. Professor Scott tried to reassure her, arguing that it was far more likely that her long-term health would suffer if she stopped flupentixol and ended up having a further relapse of depression. But something had shifted, and Emily was not convinced. Once Professor Scott accepted that she was determined to stop flupentixol, he advised caution and regular reviews by her local psychiatrist. He also warned her not to tinker with more than one drug at a time, otherwise they would not know which drug was essential when she relapsed.

Just a short time later, she read another *BMJ* article also reporting a higher mortality, but this time for patients taking benzodiazepines and/or the Z-drugs like the zolpidem she was taking to help her sleep. Once again, Professor Scott tried to reassure her, reminding her how insomnia was part of her relapse signature. Although Emily acknowledged the logic in his argument, she hadn't suffered any ill effects from stopping flupentixol and felt better, much more awake and alert during the day. However, she found it wasn't easy to sleep as she weaned herself off regular zolpidem and Emily made sure she kept some in reserve, just in case she had a particularly bad night.

Professor Scott always had Emily's best interests at heart and wanted all his patients to do well. Yet she felt conflicted by the repeated warnings of relapse if she didn't comply with the prescribed drug regimen. She did not want to be sentenced to unpleasant and potentially life-threatening adverse effects, not to mention unsatisfying sex for the rest of her life.

The high dose of venlafaxine, put Emily at risk of dangerous cardiac arrythmias particularly when combined with other drugs. She was supposed to have regular monitoring with ECGs, but the GPs didn't seem to be aware of how important this was. There was also the conflicting advice over psychotherapy; the new counsellor thought she needed to revisit the past, but Professor Scott and his team had always been adamant that it was completely unnecessary when her depression was clearly so biological in nature. While Emily's psychiatrists were decided in their own minds what was worth it to keep her well, she wondered how much her own views were part of that consideration.

## RECONSIDERATION

They had been in Northwood for over a year. Emily had survived another major relocation, and they were under intense financial pressure with the added strain of a failed house sale. As a couple they faced an uncertain future. Emily reckoned she was doing pretty well, all things considered.

Every evening Peter returned from lectures and talked about counselling. It was as if Emily was being drip-fed alternative theories to the traditional bio-medical model of psychiatry. She acknowledged her doubts that maybe doctors, psychiatrists in particular, were not quite as expert as she first thought when it came to mental illness or the problems that people faced in their everyday lives. But surely it was unconscionable that the theories of psychiatry so embedded in medical practice were not based on sound scientific evidence? Yet what she heard from Peter made sense: everyone's moods and emotions varied all the time. It wasn't unusual to experience phases or seasons in life when people might feel more upset or fed up than their 'normal', for any number of reasons. Emily wondered what distinguished a natural phenomenon from a 'diagnosis' requiring treatment with psychiatric drugs.

Peter was also studying theology and he related the cycle of emotional experiences to the writings found in the biblical book of Psalms. He was scathing of the Christian ideal of 'happy all the time' and drew attention to the suffering that was so full of meaning throughout Jewish history, as well as the early church. In his opinion, it was not feelings of depression that were the problem, rather it was the reaction to such feelings either internally within the individual or externally from a society that determined that 'one should not be feeling that way'. He thought this compounded the situation and led to an exacerbation or exaggeration of what had started off as an entirely reasonable emotion.

The penny dropped as Emily recognised how she had entered downward spirals just like this, on multiple occasions. Likewise, she saw that when she worried because she couldn't sleep, it was a sure way of making the insomnia worse. It was reassuring to recognise and accept the natural undulations of her mood and Emily no longer felt alarmed by an off-day or three.

* * *

Here are some key questions for anyone with a psychiatric diagnosis:

What were the original symptoms? Is it possible these symptoms were natural responses to circumstances, perhaps made worse by others' reactions to unexpected or heightened *emotion? If prescribed psychiatric drugs, what symptoms if any, can be attributed to the adverse effects of those drugs and/ or the withdrawal from them? Are the relationships with your healthcare team giving you more, or less, autonomy?*

# CHAPTER 26

# Watford

It was 2010 and Emily had not come across any doctor who was critical of the traditional bio-medical model of psychiatry. Despite her doubts, she remained persuaded that most of the time psychiatric diagnoses were valid and believed that treatment with drugs and ECT must be helpful. In her own case, Emily still relied on what Professor Scott had told her: that she had a severe depression characterised by relapses and remissions, caused by some kind of brain dysfunction, probably the result of a neurochemical imbalance and she needed to take antidepressant drugs for life.

## STIGMA LIVES ON

Although Emily knew that being a psychiatric patient had shaped her life and given her valuable insights which informed her compassion, she didn't think she was better than anyone else. When she wrote or spoke about her lived experience, she drew parallels with the need for continuous treatment in physical conditions and it seemed vital to redress the balance where physical suffering is taken far more seriously than the unseen consequences of emotional distress.

As she continued to witness how entrenched stigma was within the medical profession, Emily became more determined to argue the case. She despised any assertion that heightened or diminished emotional expression was a sign of weakness or character defect suffered by a select and unfortunate few. She thought patients deserved better and should never be made to suffer because of bad attitude and/or second-rate treatment delivered by the NHS. She hoped that drawing attention to the ubiquitous nature of turbulent feelings, which are part of the whole human experience, would open doors to a more compassionate health service.

The Banchory church had been the closest Emily had come to a 'mental-illness friendly' Christian community. But in the main, little had changed within the Protestant church. Christianity was supposed to be a religion based on love and yet sympathy towards those suffering with emotional problems was in short supply. It was not uncommon to hear of churchgoers who admitted to feeling down, depressed, or anxious, but were given unwarranted opinions on how their spiritual lives were lacking, rather than the compassionate response they had hoped for. It was always worse for those with formal psychiatric diagnoses, and especially for psychosis or schizophrenia; the belief in demonic possession and the involvement of the devil still persisted even in the twenty-first century.

The ethos within charismatic and newer Protestant churches seemed particularly unbalanced; many preachers glossed over life's difficulties, hiding behind a superficial veneer posing as spirituality. Certain bible verses were taken completely out of context and interpreted to support their current dogma.

Emily was curious about why Christians were expected to put a uniformly positive spin on their experiences. It seemed that consciously deterring people from authentically expressing themselves, was not just damaging to individuals but also to those around them. Peter and Emily concluded that the church needed urgent education on the subject of mental health, and they explored ideas on how to share their experiences. Emily longed to express her solidarity with those who felt excluded and belittled; it motivated her to write another book. *A Thorn in My Mind: Mental Illness, Stigma and The Church* was published in 2012. The first memoir had had a limited impact on her own profession, but she hoped that her fellow Christians might be more receptive.

Since I no longer adhere to the same beliefs in fundamentalist, evangelical Christianity that I had at the time of writing, and I was still convinced of the rightness of the bio-medical diagnosis of depression, I have subsequently requested that the book be withdrawn. But whatever the root causes of people's problems, I continue to support the premise that every individual who suffers symptoms related to their mental health, should be treated with respect, kindness, and compassion, especially in the Christian church which is supposed to model loving one's neighbour.

## PEER SUPPORT

Emily helped launch a support group for those with mental health problems in her community and regularly visited a friend who had been admitted to the local psychiatric unit. It was horrifying to witness how little had changed and it was uncanny how little effort the staff made to hide their disrespect and punitive attitudes towards their patients. Emily wrote to the unit's management when she saw staff demeaning a patient who had spilt their food. The unit's response was to ban visitors from the dining area. Emily vowed that she would never allow herself to be admitted to a psychiatric ward again. As an elected patient-governor at the Trust where she was still receiving outpatient care, Emily volunteered to take part in the 'Recovery College'. It was abundantly clear that there was still a long way to go to eliminate bad practice and change staff attitudes, but at least they were trying.

## WORK PREPARATIONS

When the Banchory house sold, Peter and Emily bought a place in Watford. A few weeks later, their washing machine, dishwasher, oven, and car broke down simultaneously. It shook Emily out of complacency, and she knew she had to start earning again.

Emily had stopped flupentixol completely without ill effect and only took zolpidem occasionally. She became convinced that the remaining 'symptoms' such as emotional numbness and feelings of unreality were adverse effects of the two antidepressants; nonetheless she continued to take them religiously. Since these experiences had always been interpreted as evidence of depression, she simply stopped reporting them.

The time seemed right to overcome her fear of relapse, which had been so successfully instilled into her by the well-intentioned psychiatric profession. Increasingly confident after surviving yet another upheaval of moving house, but unwilling to risk disaster, Emily promised to take it one step at a time.

The move to Watford meant another catchment area and another new psychiatrist. This one was perplexed by Emily's history of depression, as well as Professor Scott's advice to continue prophylaxis with such high doses of venlafaxine and trazodone, especially given how well Emily was. He arranged to see her for one further appointment before writing a letter to support her re-employment as a doctor.

Emily was not yet confident enough to contemplate reducing or stopping the two remaining antidepressants. It seemed like the prognosis of certain relapse had become embedded in her psyche. She couldn't risk putting their future in jeopardy while trying to return to work in a stressful job, and she resigned herself to the fact that she was saddled with adverse effects and robbed of an enjoyable sex life.

The clinical director of the A&E department at Watford General Hospital, was cautious but willing to consider Emily's desire to work in Emergency Medicine again. However, the administrative machine ground slowly – it took until spring 2013 for Emily to be granted Occupational Health clearance and given an honorary contract to spend time in A&E as an unpaid clinical observer. But the benefits system only permitted a maximum of sixteen hours a week for any activity, paid or voluntary which could be classed as work, and benefits were still a vital source of financial support. Emily decided to test the waters before she surrendered them.

## WATFORD A&E

Despite the years that had passed since she last worked in Emergency Medicine, the return to A&E as a clinical observer felt far more comfortable than working on a psychiatric ward. There was a new universal 'bare below the elbows' rule, which left Emily feeling slightly self-conscious. Eagle-eyed medics never miss a thing, and it took a while before she was confident enough to talk about the elephant in the room, and explain the scars on her arms from decades ago.

It was a great day when the clinical director said that Emily could do some paid shifts as a locum doctor.

When Emily called the benefits office to surrender her incapacity benefit, a woman asked her how she felt. "I'm so happy to be able to earn a living once again," Emily replied, and she meant it.

Admittedly she did have some mixed feelings; it was tough to look back at where she was, prior to the move to Scotland. She had been a specialist registrar in the busiest A&E on the south coast, with lots of responsibility and a good deal of autonomy. Undoubtedly, she had a lot of catching up to do as she refreshed her skills and updated her knowledge that had become rusty during the intervening years. Then finally the day came when she was invited to apply for a registrar post at Watford General Hospital. Emily still remained cautious, working part-time and only slowly building up the number of hours she worked.

## CHURCH SCRUPLES

During 2015, Peter and Emily became increasingly uncomfortable with their church. One Sunday during the sermon, the pastor denounced a book, *Love Wins* by Rob Bell and it was subsequently banned from the local Christian bookstore where Emily's own book had been a bestseller. This piqued Emily's curiosity, and she ordered it online. She found the alternative interpretations of the bible and different views about the Christian faith refreshing. Peter and Emily dropped out of the Sunday church meetings and instead joined a group of volunteers who provided breakfast for those who were homeless. Shortly afterwards, the church leaders met with Peter and Emily; they mutually agreed to part company, because they did not share the same views.

At the Sunday breakfasts, they met an extraordinary man called Dave who had been homeless for years. He realised what an impact modern living had on everyone's carbon footprint, which greatly contributed to global warming. He has remained a good friend ever since.

## DENVER DECISIONS

While on holiday in Denver visiting their son, Harry, Peter and Emily started thinking more about their long-term future.

Although Emily enjoyed working back in A&E, she had hoped there would be the opportunity to complete her postgraduate training and become a consultant. But there didn't seem any realistic possibility of advancing her career in her current job. She desperately wanted to improve the care of patients with mental health problems, but she had discovered how difficult it was to significantly influence the culture without the benefit of being in a senior role within the medical hierarchy.

Perhaps it was this growing discontent in several areas of their lives that drove Peter and Emily to make an incredibly bold decision. As the parents of an American citizen, they had a legal right to apply for permanent residency in the USA. They both decided to leave their jobs, sell their house, and move to Denver while they were still young enough to re-establish themselves in work. Immediately Emily set about preparing for the notoriously difficult USMLE (United States Medical Licensing Examinations), undeterred by the fact that she would need to do the intensive three-year hospital residency programme to become a board-certified Emergency Physician. She still naively trusted that God was in control, optimistic that life had a habit of working out one way or another.

Emily's confidence in the robustness of her recovery had grown. She still maintained contact with Professor Scott, respected his opinion and appreciated the care he had given her, but was increasingly doubtful of his gloomy prognosis of relapse. The impending emigration to America was the stimulus Emily needed to start weaning down the doses of venlafaxine and trazodone.

## LEAVING

The estate agents were confident of a quick sale when the house went on the market, and they soon had a buyer. Then a week later, the surprise results of the Brexit vote were announced, and property prices plummeted. Their buyer pulled out, unable to sell their own property. This same scenario repeated itself time and again, while mortgage offers failed, or the chain broke down. But Peter and Emily had already bought their plane tickets, resigned from their jobs, and given most of their furniture and belongings away. The personal effects they wanted to take to Denver were in storage waiting to be shipped once they found a place to live. The house price fell, their assets dwindling away before their eyes and they wondered how long they would be forced to live out of the three suitcases they had left to take with them.

In August 2016, Peter and Emily spent their last weekend in their Watford house with their friend, Dave. As they sat together in the garden, he told them more about the challenge to slow down global warming. Emily was alarmed at how air travel in particular was such a huge contributor to global carbon emissions. Climate change hadn't been high on their list of priorities and yet Dave did not berate them. He quietly shared his thoughts with honesty and gentleness without forcing his views on them. Emily thought the evangelicals could learn a thing or two from him. It was the one and only time they managed to persuade him to take a bed for the night. The irony of the situation was not lost on them.

It was hard to say goodbye to their family, even though they knew that it was physically impossible to live on the same continent as all of them. Peter and Emily may have thought they were flying away from trouble, but it wasn't long before they discovered they were sorely mistaken.

\* \* \*

*Please do not be overly surprised if you find doctors who are still largely ignorant about the withdrawal symptoms associated with reducing or stopping antidepressants or other psychiatric drugs. It* is urgent that the medical profession becomes sufficiently educated to help those patients who want to stop their medication do so safely, and reduce the risk of harmful, long-term withdrawal syndromes.

If you are thinking of stopping or changing psychiatric drugs, please seek help from your doctor. (There are some resources in the appendix.)

# CHAPTER 27

# Emigration

When they arrived in Denver, Peter and Emily were offered temporary accommodation in the basement of a friend's house. It was an adventure to be living in a bedsit – a throwback to when they were first married.

## IMMIGRATION MEDICAL

As healthy adults, Emily hadn't paid much attention to the list of prohibited medical conditions which could invalidate their application for permanent residency. They had paid for relevant blood tests and immunisations and all that remained was the appointment with a doctor certified to do immigration medicals.

A few days before, Emily was shocked and alarmed to find that any past history of 'harm to self or others' was on the list of prohibited conditions. While a history of violence seemed understandable, the discovery that previous episodes of self-harm might thwart her chance of getting the precious green card (permanent residency) was exceptionally worrying.

Even though the last act of self-harm was almost a decade ago, Emily wasn't prepared to take any chances. She collated all her recent medical information including the letters about her psychiatric care, and emailed both Professor Scott and the clinical director from her previous job in Watford, requesting validation of her recovery. They both replied immediately with statements testifying to her fitness for work and that she had not posed a 'risk' to herself for many years, and had *never* been a risk to others.

On the day of the immigration medical, Peter and Emily arrived for their appointment at a primary care facility and joined the crowd of people in the waiting room. They were called through together and introduced to a physician assistant (PA). She addressed questions to Peter first, while simultaneously checking off tick boxes on a form in front of her. Emily assumed that this was a preliminary interview before they saw the doctor. Then the PA turned her attention to Emily and did the same thing, before dismissing them back to the waiting room.

A short while later, the receptionist called them over and handed Peter a sealed envelope containing the completed medical reports. She explained it was their responsibility to send this on to the immigration authorities. Thankfully Peter had paid extra to retain copies of the report for their own records. Emily was surprised that they hadn't actually seen a doctor and hadn't been asked for any evidence of their medical histories. As they were leaving, she quickly scanned through her own medical report. On the top in bold was a prominent warning that giving false information was a violation of immigration law and would lead to immediate deportation.

Then Emily spotted the obvious error. The box, 'no history of mental illness', had been checked. She rushed back to the reception desk and knocked on the glass partition and asked to see the doctor. The receptionist rolled her eyes and in a bored voice, replied, "The assessment has been done, there's no need to see anyone else."

Emily tried to explain that there had been a mistake. The receptionist shrugged and told her there were no more appointments. When Emily insisted, she was told they'd just have to wait.

For the next hour, Emily felt sick, trembling slightly, aware of the curiosity on the faces of others in the waiting room. Eventually Emily was called through and met the same PA again. This time the PA had a grim expression on her face and pursed her lips as Emily explained that she had been depressed in the past and self-harmed but was now completely well. The PA accused Emily of withholding information. Emily apologised for the misunderstanding, explaining that she thought they would be seeing the doctor. (She could hardly point out that the PA hadn't actually asked her whether she had any past history of mental illness.)

Emily volunteered that she was fully prepared to answer any questions about her mental health and offered the PA her folder containing all the letters, statements, and other documents. The PA waved it away without a glance and once again dismissed Emily back to the waiting room without asking any further details about what she had just disclosed.

Another hour passed, and Emily sat sweating despite the chill of the air-conditioning. Finally, the receptionist handed over another sealed envelope and a new copy of the report, but this time they stood there while Emily meticulously read it through. It felt like a punch to the stomach when she spotted a cross in the box 'currently at risk of harm to self and others'.

Emily's imagination went into free fall as in a moment she saw how it had all been in vain. Peter would be left here in Denver, while she would be deported, having failed the immigration medical. Her tongue stuck to the roof of her mouth, as she demanded that she must see the doctor who they had paid to perform their immigration medical examinations. The receptionist glared at them. "The report has already been changed once and *this* is the final version."

Emily pleaded with her, asking that she at least give her documents to the physician in charge. The receptionist was defiant. "No," she said.

Risking everything, Emily refused to leave and thankfully just at that moment, the PA walked in, wondering what the fuss was about. Her brow wrinkled, and she frowned until Emily pointed to the problem on the form, then she broke into laughter. "Oh, I must have checked the wrong box."

Without hesitation she agreed to put it right and let Emily confirm that it had been done correctly. She selected the option: 'previous history of harm to self or others but no current risk' and this time she invited Emily to instruct her on what to write in the comments section which up until now had been left blank.

They never did see the doctor paid to evaluate their health. None of Emily's supporting documents were ever looked at, and Emily was never asked any questions about her current state of mind. What had just transpired could not possibly constitute a valid risk assessment of her mental health.

When they got home and described their ordeal to their landlord, he shook his head and sighed. "Welcome to America," he said.

## HEADACHE

One day, Emily suddenly developed the worst headache she had ever had. In the ER, the CT scan and lumbar puncture were all normal, but she was admitted with extremely high blood pressure. Once discharged, a couple from the church came down to their basement room to pray for her. They were convinced that the spirit world was real and thought that Emily's headache was a sign of demonic attack. With authoritative voices, they invoked the power of God and rebuked the devil. Strangely Emily felt better and was able to get some sleep. They advised her to quote scripture regularly and 'resist the devil'. They were such lovely people, nonetheless it felt unnerving. It was not the first time they had come across such fervent belief, but it seemed more extreme.

## STRESSES

Undoubtedly the first few months in Denver were very stressful; the house in Watford remained unsold and their savings were slowly being whittled away. Emily didn't know if she would be subjected to further evaluation following the immigration medical. Peter and Emily had already invested heavily in their emigration plans, and if Emily continued to pursue the USMLE (United States Medical Licensing Exams), there would be further financial outlay. There was an expensive entry fee for each step of the exam, and she had to fly to one of the specialist centres to take the clinical skills part. Her success was incumbent on performing well in Step 1, widely acknowledged as the most difficult part of the exam. The statistics were hardly promising – only fifty per cent of FMGs (Foreign Medical Graduates) passed Step 1 on the first attempt. Suddenly, Emily felt her age, and wondered how she could compete against those from American medical schools in their twenties and thirties, when answering multiple choice questions during the eight- and nine-hour long examinations.

## JOB PROSPECTS

Studying had been arduous, but it all seemed worthwhile on the day the results came out. Emily was delighted with the smart certificate granting her eligibility to apply for the hospital residency programmes via the national computer matching service, ERAS. But when it came time to enter her data on ERAS, it repeatedly bounced back with a message to seek further advice from the programme, and every time she tried to get in contact, she could never reach anyone.

Emily tried it out with other residency programmes throughout Colorado and then in other states, but the same thing happened. It was a terrible shock when she finally uncovered the problem was one of red tape.

Despite the numerous documents she had submitted including all the dates and results of every stage of her medical school training, there was no mention of a vital bit of information that stipulated that in most states, including Colorado, she had to have left medical school during the previous five years. The fact that she qualified years earlier completely excluded her from the application process. She looked through every email, letter and webpage, and had not come across this limitation before. She was absolutely devastated. Some years later, Emily discovered there were a few exceptions to this rule in some states, but there was certainly no easy way of finding this out.

Ironically, their house had just sold, and their shipment arrived from England. Peter and Emily's work permits were granted and without any further problems, the green cards arrived in the post. It was such a strange time and Emily didn't know what to think. All she knew was that finding work had become the top priority.

Peter found a temporary job, using his IT/admin skills. As Emily scoured the internet, she was excited to find a 'non-profit' called the Spring Institute, which helped to find jobs for FMGs (Foreign Medical Graduates). She drove downtown to an appointment with one of the caseworkers. Nigel ushered her through to a small room at the back of what looked like a crowded and run-down office. They sat down and Emily handed him a copy of her CV, as requested. However, Nigel didn't mirror her hopeful demeanour. He scowled as he took a pen from his pocket and struck a diagonal line across every page of Emily's CV. With little emotion he said, "The only good thing about your résumé, is that English is your first language."

It was a warm, spring day and despite the blue sky visible through the open window, it felt as though the world had clouded over. Surely, she should be accustomed to receiving bad news by now. Nigel was firing questions at her, but it was as if she couldn't hear him. Finally, her attention returned. "Have you thought about training to be a care home worker or a phlebotomist?" Nigel asked.

He handed her a sheet of paper, listing potential jobs which had a loose connection to the world of medicine. "You need to convince the employer that your interest in a position is not just because you can't work as a doctor," he warned.

A few days later, Emily plucked up the courage to call the Spring Institute again and she was invited to a group session on résumé writing. There were about eight others of various ages, sat around the table and Emily was the only woman. Apparently, Nigel had moved on, and Emily hoped that his imminent departure was the reason for his pessimism.

Trixie was altogether different, a bright and cheerful lady. She asked each doctor to introduce themselves. Emily was the only one who had already completed the exams. Trixie advised them not to waste any money on applications for medical posts in Colorado; they had not accepted a single foreign graduate onto any residency programme for over thirty years. She encouraged them all to pursue alternative employment.

The rest of the workshop was devoted to résumé writing. No wonder Emily's British CV was not acceptable. It bore no resemblance to the single page résumé, which they were encouraged to write. To Emily it seemed to be an exercise in self-aggrandisement, and she certainly had no means to demonstrate how much money she had made or saved for the NHS during her career. The Spring Institute did indeed help immigrant medical professionals to find work, but while they remained in Colorado it would not be as doctors.

But the bad news didn't end there. To get a job in even basic healthcare-related activities like phlebotomy required an American qualification. Emily thought it was bad enough that she had to retake her driving test. Everything she considered required more training at further cost. How ironic it all seemed; there was no exemption even though Emily had passed the advanced American medical licensing examinations, and her British degrees did not count either.

But Emily was unwilling to give up yet and pursued every contact she could find. She met doctors and academics who worked at the medical school and university. She met doctors disillusioned with the system who had set up businesses. Everyone was friendly and expressed outrage at the absurdity of the situation, as well as their admiration for her enormous achievement in passing the USMLE at this stage in her career. She followed up on many suggestions and potential opportunities, but they all led up blind alleys.

However, Emily did make exceptions; she was not prepared to work for the 'dark side' – for medical insurance companies. There were numerous advertisements for doctors to work in non-clinical roles, but she had already experienced first-hand, the work of doctors who screened insurance claims, arguing how clients failed to meet small print criteria in order to refuse them. Likewise, she had no appetite to work for pharmaceutical companies promoting the sales of their drugs.

Again, Emily returned to the list of alternative careers from the Spring Institute and decided to apply for training as a medical coder which at least seemed neutral, well remunerated and could be done from home. The course director gave her a call, interested in her application. After Emily explained her situation, the director responded: "I don't normally say this to applicants," she said, "but I strongly advise you not to pay for this course. You will be bored and frustrated as a medical coder. Do something else."

Emily appreciated her honesty, but it felt like she had come to the end of the line. Her medical career was well and truly over, and she was underqualified without American college degrees, and at the same time overqualified in terms of experience.

Peter, likewise, was very much in the same boat. While Emily was still reeling from the extreme disappointment, she had to congratulate herself that she had survived a formidable amount of stress without any detriment to her mental health. She resigned herself to the reality that she had wasted a considerable amount of time and money in pursuit of an American medical career; it was time to move on.

## MORE DECISIONS

Long-term relapse prevention was not covered by American health insurance and so the cost of psychotropic drugs like venlafaxine would only be financed for the *treatment* of active psychiatric conditions. Emily had no desire to reacquire a psychiatric diagnosis just to get expensive medication paid for by the medical insurance. Besides which she wondered just why she should keep taking nasty drugs with their unpleasant adverse effects. Was it just to keep her UK psychiatrists happy? She laughed at the absurdity of it all; perhaps they should be the ones to take her antidepressants!

At church, Peter and Emily came across plenty of people with stories of trial and tribulation after a move to Denver, but Emily thought they were facing rather larger stakes, relatively late in life. Yet she still held out the hope that it wasn't too late to realise their potential, here in the land of dreams.

\* \* \*

*Hope is a very powerful antidepressant, but turmoil and difficult emotions may also be worth paying attention to. How do you feel about listening to your innermost being? Can you identify anything that can boost your levels of hope?*

# CHAPTER 28

# New directions

## ITINERANT PREACHER

Emily was convinced that God had led them to Denver, but it was the warmth of spring, along with the blue skies and the constant sunshine that lifted her spirits.

The guest preacher, a man in his late thirties, often visited Denver as part of his itinerant ministry, and was given a rousing welcome at church. It was attested that he had presided over several miraculous healings. Emily found the topic fascinating; she had heard many Christians preach about healing but had seen little evidence to support their claims of 'miracles', which were often based on events overseas. She kept an open mind, still puzzled by her own unexplained 'light experience', which had propelled her to recovery in 2001, and still remained the nearest thing to a miracle that she had ever come across.

The preacher was entertaining and enthusiastic. There was a dramatic pause before he asked if the church wanted to see a miracle. Emily's heart sank. He used a common tactic she had seen plenty of times before, asking the congregation to raise their hands if they suffered with a common ailment. It was a no-brainer, of course there was going to be at least one person in a group of this size.

The preacher took the microphone with him as he approached a young woman and asked Karina a bit more about her symptoms. He gestured dramatically as he asked everyone to gather round and switch on their phones to record a miracle. "As you can see," the preacher told the onlookers, "the reason for her back pain is that her legs are not the same length."

There was nothing to see. Then he instructed a bold and authoritative prayer to be said. The person sitting next to Karina obliged. "Be healed in Jesus's name." Karina gave a little shudder and the preacher was excited. "Did you see it? Did you see her leg grow?"

Karina was honest when he asked her how she felt. She said she didn't know since she didn't actually have back pain before the prayer. The preacher didn't seem to mind; he insisted that a healing miracle had taken place. The church meeting was drawing to a close, and it was announced that baskets would be left near the exits, so that people could give the preacher a 'love offering', on their way out.

Emily was concerned and went to talk to one of the church leaders. She had not seen any miracle. The leader shrugged. "I'm not a doctor, so I cannot comment."

Not satisfied, Emily waited until most people had left before she went to speak to the preacher. She explained her medical background and as diplomatically as she could, she challenged what had happened. He responded by accusing Emily that she did not believe in the healing power of God. Emily countered by telling him her own story of the light experience which terminated her depression. He wasn't impressed and Emily realised that there was no point in pursuing the matter further.

Later, she reflected on how sad it was that many itinerant preachers' incomes depended on the donations they received from their preaching tours. She suspected the talk of 'living by faith' was very much dependent on their performance in church. Perhaps the truth was that they lived off the kindness and gullibility of Christians who were drawn into these fundamentalist church circles.

Ironically, she knew someone who had suffered great pain and disability from legs of different lengths, but the Almighty hadn't shown them any miraculous favours; instead they had to undergo painful corrective surgery.

## CHRISTIAN HEALING

As it was, Emily was in complete awe of the complexity of the human body. She saw no conflict in believing that a God who had created people who healed naturally every day, would be perfectly capable of doing miracles. What she struggled with, was the inequity and injustice that is so apparent when so many people the world over desperately needed some divine intervention. She tried to let go of her qualms and remember how many genuine and sensible Christians testified to seeing extraordinary healings and miracles.

However, this incident left her feeling unhappy with church. Peter and Emily were still without permanent employment and urgently needed somewhere else to live. They had burned their bridges and returning to the UK seemed as difficult as staying in America.

## FINDING A FUTURE

The next most pressing concern was finding somewhere to live, before rushing into any final decisions over their long-term future. Peter and Emily stumbled across some very reasonably priced apartments in Windsor Gardens, the first purpose-built village for 'active, older adults' over the age of fifty. The apartments were large, built around a central golf course. There was a community building with swimming pools, bar, restaurant, theatre, and library. When they went back a second time, they realised that if they bought an apartment outright, then the monthly community charge would be less than paying rent.

Before she left England, Emily had joked that if all else failed, at least she could clean toilets. What was said in jest was about to become reality when Emily was offered a job at Holy Helpers (HH), a centre for the homeless and gave her some much-needed peace of mind.

By June 2017, Emily had started work at HH and she sat with Peter by the outdoor pool at Windsor Gardens, dangling their feet in the cool water. Their new two-bed apartment was unusual because it hadn't been renovated, but they weren't bothered by the dated fixtures and fittings in the kitchen and bathrooms. They planned to modernise the apartment once they were settled, and their finances were more secure.

## TRAZODONE WITHDRAWAL

Having weathered so much in the previous year, Emily remained well. She was still taking trazodone, having weaned down to 30mg from the original 300mg. However, it was disappointing when she tried to stop it completely – she developed a ghastly feeling that her legs needed to move which felt intolerable. Severe rebound insomnia accompanied the terrible restlessness and she had gone without sleep for seventy-two hours. Emily restarted the trazodone. Fortunately, the symptoms settled when she resumed the medication.

Still very ignorant about withdrawal syndromes or how to taper them safely, Emily hadn't realised that 30mg was still far too high a dose to stop the drug precipitously. Thankfully her new GP was happy to cite 'restless leg syndrome' as the reason for the prescription, but Emily still hoped to stop it at a later date. She was having more success at weaning down to tiny doses of venlafaxine. When the 'electric shock' symptoms intensified, she remembered her experiences from fifteen years earlier and cut the venlafaxine tablets into tiny little slivers. She carried bits around with her in a plastic bag, to take any time the symptoms became intolerable. It wasn't measured and it wasn't scientific as she slowly prolonged the period between each dose, leaving it as long as she could before taking a fragment of a pill. It took months but at last, she had completely stopped venlafaxine.

Emily started to feel more alive even before she had completely weaned off venlafaxine; she no longer felt numb, and the world felt different. It was as though she had been living life in two dimensions and now, she was whole, back in a three-dimensional world.

Admittedly, it could be alarming to feel such intense emotion, but more often she appreciated the fact that she could feel so deeply for the first time in years, and she even relished her new ability to cry loud and long with real tears. Emily also delighted in the experience of sheer joy and exhilaration in a way she had been deprived of for so long. Furthermore, Emily's sex life was back and at last, she felt like a whole person once again.

## NEW HOME

Peter and Emily furnished their new apartment from second-hand sales and were delighted with the quality they could buy at very reasonable prices. Emily joined a writers' group, they met their neighbours and forged new friendships within the community. Now the future seemed more secure, they booked their first trip back to visit family in October.

Life had definitely improved but Emily decided to get some counselling to process the disappointments and stress from the preceding year. It was at this point that she met Barb, which is where this book began but it is certainly not the end of the story.

* * *

*There is a balance to be made for people who have been taking psychiatric drugs for a long time, between continuing with adverse effects and the risks of potential withdrawal problems. I hope that you can make the right decision for yourself without feeling any pressure either way.*

# CHAPTER 29

# Counselling

Barb was unashamedly a Christian counsellor and based herself at a large local church where Peter and Emily intended to go for services. Peter tried to warn Emily that it might limit her independence as a therapist, but Barb reassured Emily that confidentiality was paramount.

Barb had furnished her counselling room with soft covered armchairs and a comfortable sofa, alongside a combination of candles and plants; it was relaxing, almost luxurious, very different from the NHS, but so were the prices involved. Emily declined her offer to open the sessions with prayer.

## BACKGROUND

At first, Barb hadn't seemed very sympathetic when Emily told her about the relationship difficulties that had resulted over differences in opinion on Christian issues. It felt like Barb was being dismissive when she assured Emily that God would handle any injustice. But the dynamics rapidly changed when Barb asked more about Emily's background and life history. As outlined in Chapter 1, Emily explained how the UK psychiatrists had advised against further exploration of her childhood difficulties and regurgitated their reasoning that her early life events had given her 'vulnerability factors' but had not caused the depression.

When Barb dropped the bombshell by suggesting that she hadn't been depressed at all back in 1994, Emily was so astonished she didn't know what to say. But before the session ended, Barb challenged Emily over her willingness to change. She asked her to return the following week with notes on who she thought she was, and the benefits and drawbacks of keeping her current identity versus those of changing the views she had of herself.

## IDENTITY QUESTION

Back at home, Emily pondered some more over the reasons Barb could come to such a radically different conclusion within such a short space of time. It had opened up the possibility that she had endured years of treatment at the hands of psychiatry for no good reason. Emily realised that if she was going to take Barb's therapy seriously, she would need to re-evaluate her identity, the books she had written and the many times she had spoken about her experiences of depression. Barb's interpretation of events intrigued Emily and she decided to persevere for at least a few more sessions; it seemed refreshing that as a Christian, Barb would at least understand her faith.

During the next few appointments, Barb gathered the details of Emily's early life and background, much of which is written in earlier chapters. Barb was easily the first person to identify just how damaging Emily's boarding school experience had been. She also saw strong parallels between Emily's time at boarding school and the hospital admissions and recognised how re-traumatising it would have been. When Emily described how she had related the very same stories about her childhood and described the very same distress, many times over during the seven-year nightmare, Barb just slowly shook her head. Barb's conclusions definitely made sense and for the first time since she originally sought help in 1994, Emily felt that someone was really listening. It had taken over twenty-three years.

Emily was painfully aware that she did not have great relationships with some of her close family members, but over the sessions, Barb was able to bring a new perspective. She asked Emily to take a step back and see herself through the eyes of her family. It was very uncomfortable as Barb painted a picture of how she thought the family saw her, but Barb's insights seemed accurate, and Emily was filled with remorse.

Barb thought Emily was the 'strong' one with a forceful personality when she first met Peter, especially when she thought she was right. Not only was she opinionated, but she was also intolerant of her own emotions, unable to show her weakness – the persona that enabled her to survive boarding school.

Emily admitted that she *wanted* Peter to be dominant in their relationship because it was how the gender roles had been portrayed during her upbringing. Subsequently this was reinforced by the church dogma which stated that the husband must be the head of the household and the wage earner. Embedded in the church wedding vows was the agreement to 'honour and obey'. Peter loved Emily and wasn't trying to change her. But Emily desperately wanted to feel she belonged in the church community, and it motivated her failed attempts to become a quiet, submissive wife while she simultaneously tried to deny her own character and personality.

When she started work, Emily had reverted and tried to be 'strong' which was necessary given the predominantly masculine and bullying culture of medicine at the time. Once Emily was diagnosed as 'mentally ill', it was as if the coin had flipped and she became weak, feeble, totally dependent on others, and unable to fend for herself.

The children would have grown up with their strong and reliable mother until she became ill. They found it scary when it all changed. They would have been constantly worried that their Mum might never come out of hospital and afraid that she might die. After the 'healing' in 2001, suddenly and without warning, Emily flipped back into strong mode which was particularly unsettling for the children. Later, in 2006, after a period when Emily had kept her feelings hidden, it was yet another sudden change when she collapsed in a heap and went back into hospital. Barb thought the children subconsciously wondered whether they could ever trust their Mum again. She surmised that they weren't reassured by her subsequent recovery. How could they be sure it wouldn't happen again? They probably didn't like her as a person who couldn't cope with life, any more than Emily liked herself. Although she had intended to protect her family by hiding her feelings, all it had done was increase their fears.

## CHALLENGE

In Denver, Peter and Emily faced all sorts of difficulties and this time Emily had her fluctuating emotions on display, which naturally confused and/or provoked anxiety within her family. But Barb's insights never came without a challenge. She was brutally honest as she reiterated that if Emily held on to self-pity and regret, she would inadvertently push those she loved further away from her, and Emily would perceive this as rejection, a cycle which would never lead to resolution.

Barb seemed to have hit the nail on the head as she outlined how Emily had compounded, if not created further difficulties within the family. It was hard not to feel ashamed, and Emily felt afraid that she would never get it right, always prone to repeat her previous mistakes which she had demonstrated with tedious regularity since their arrival in Denver.

## COPING STRATEGY

Barb had more insights to share about how Emily's character developed, and she felt an urgent need to get to grips with her well-established but maladaptive coping mechanisms.

Emily started 'working hard' for the first time in senior school, hoping to get sent home. Her goal was thwarted, but because she pushed herself to study, it unlocked secondary gains and academic success which led to much longed for affirmation and also coincided with the bonding of good friendships. This was Emily's sentinel experience of 'strong' mode, and she learnt guts, grind, determination, and perseverance. The benefits were obvious – Emily had tasted success, admiration, and approval. The problem was not that Emily worked hard, it was that when stressed, her response was to work harder, and this became unsustainable and led to burn-out. Undoubtedly this was an accurate description of what happened back in 1994 and Emily was more convinced than ever that her original diagnosis had been wrong, not just during the seven-year period of treatment-resistant depression, but for everything that followed since.

## RELIGIOUS SOLUTION

The last counsellor Emily had really appreciated was Graham, who had consistently reassured Emily of her self-worth. Barb's therapy in contrast seemed harsh, but Emily thought she was probably right. Barb recognised that Emily had grown up without believing she was loved unconditionally, and she never felt truly accepted for who she was. While this resonated as true, Barb's solutions were harder to embrace.

Barb encouraged Emily to become totally 'dependent on God', trust him and let him 'take all her feelings of guilt, regret and anger'. The consistent Christian teaching that she had been born in sin and only made acceptable because she had been redeemed by Christ, was all the confirmation Emily needed that her core self was fundamentally flawed. Barb did not contradict this view and session by session she continued to promote the idea that the breakthrough would come only when Emily relied on God for approval, acceptance, and love. Barb endorsed the reality of this 'relationship with God' as she told Emily this was how she had found freedom for herself, as she became certain of God's love for her.

Although Barb's insights were valuable, she didn't spot another well-developed pattern as she assumed the role of 'expert' in Emily's life. Emily couldn't see it either and instead felt a tremendous pressure to conform, as she deferred to Barb's 'special' knowledge. Emily genuinely wanted to experience this deep connection with God that so many Christians described and though she tried to develop this elusive 'relationship with God', she didn't get any nearer to the utopian state of peace and tranquillity.

## CHURCH IDEOLOGY

The church had their own jargon, much like a regional dialect. Friends and fellow churchgoers were passionate about their faith and dedicated their whole lives to the church ideology. They said they knew God loved them and they loved worshipping him. They talked about 'hearing God' and spoke endlessly about answers to their prayers. But Emily's expectations didn't match her experience. She had questions. Was this for real?

While the Christians appeared completely genuine, she still wanted to see the evidence for all their talk. They seemed just as anxious, just as money loving, just as inconsiderate and selfish as anyone else she met. She couldn't help wondering whether she was witnessing a mass delusion or worse still, a huge 'scam'.

There were plenty of church leaders who lived off the goodwill of their congregations. Many churchgoers paid a tithe of at least ten per cent of their income before tax, straight into the church funds. Christianity was a commodity saturated with Christian books, Christian conferences, and courses about Christian living. It seemed that the church leaders' wisdom did not come for free. Many preachers made a career for themselves, travelling all over the world, speaking. Christianity had certainly become a marketable product.

## THE FICTION

Emily thought that the only way she could test it out, was to give herself fully to God. She wrote passionate prayers, read her bible, did her best to be fully engaged in all the church meetings and activities. She presented herself for prayer on numerous occasions. She was equally as dedicated as anyone else and could certainly imagine the answers a good God might give. But still she couldn't shake the feeling that she was witnessing a parody of the emperor's new clothes. There was plenty of talk about God acting in a certain way, claims of miracles, claims that they could see angels in the room... Yet Emily felt little and saw nothing.

Perhaps she was tired; after all, as a couple, Peter and Emily had been through a lot. They had moved into a completely different culture, 'separated by a common language'. Maybe Barb was right, it was Emily's propensity to *not* follow God, that was the real cause of their problems. Barb kept cajoling her, saying that God needed to be the centre of her attention and warned her that there was still a lot of 'spiritual' work to do, in order to heal from the past.

## HEIGHTENED EMOTION

Emily had recently stopped venlafaxine, although she was still on a low dose of trazodone. She had never talked in such depth with any counsellor or therapist about significant issues from the past, without the numbing influence of antidepressants. She was also trying to manage the increased intensity of raw emotion that is so common during withdrawal and at times Emily felt extremely vulnerable. Barb was often visibly moved as Emily shared some of her most distressing memories. Emily found it comforting when Barb sat beside her and at times held her hand, a complete faux pas with most therapists.

Emily fully appreciated that much of the pain caused by her childhood experiences remained unresolved and also agreed with Barb's presumption that the influences from that time were considerable. There was progress and increasingly Emily was able to reframe some of her most significant and painful memories; the freedom came as they lost their hold over her. It was empowering to know that whatever she had been through in the past, had shaped the person she was today.

Barb softened in Emily's eyes when she suggested that she had lacked role models during her adolescence. Her family relationships at that time had been very superficial. Barb also thought that Emily probably developed an idealised view of Christian family life during her brief stays with her uncle. Peter and Emily married young and once she graduated from medical school, they'd been heavily influenced and indoctrinated by immature church leaders. She reminded Emily that she never knew what went on behind closed doors; she had believed a fantasy reinforced by church leaders who had seemed able to hide their own weakness and ineptitude behind a mask of religiosity. It was as though Emily's long list of failings had shortened a bit and maybe Barb's religious views weren't quite as dogmatic as she had come to fear.

Peter and Emily were much more settled, and Emily now had a variety of friends from different walks of life, including fellow writers from both the Denver branch of the National League of American Pen Women and the Aurora Writers' Group. Although there were times when counselling brought up issues that were complex and confusing, Emily was certainly enjoying life more and also found great solace in her new job.

\* \* \*

*Emily benefited greatly from counselling, but Barb wasn't a perfect fit. Are you seeing a counsellor or psychotherapist? There are many different paths to meaningful breakthrough including art, dance, drama, music, writing or another modality in addition to or instead of talking therapy. What is important for each person is finding what is right for them.*

# CHAPTER 30

# Working with the homeless

Emily found work helpful for a number of reasons. It definitely distracted her from her own problems and put them in perspective. The homeless people were raw, and ironically Emily felt more at home with people who had nothing to hide. She identified with their vulnerability and knowing her own escape from the trials and traumas of life gave her hope for their future.

## COMMUNITY CENTRE

Holy Helpers (HH) was a non-profit organisation whose purpose was to help homeless men make good and return to mainstream society. Emily's job title, 'emergency services coordinator', sounded important but belied reality. Most of her colleagues were young idealists, good people from church backgrounds who wanted to help. They earned little more than minimum wage, worked six days a week on fixed shifts, often working every weekend. Typical for the USA, employees received two weeks annual leave and a maximum of five days sick leave. The challenge for those working directly with the homeless clientele (guests), was to retain their humanity and kindness, without suffering burn-out or compassion fatigue.

Emily worked on the early shift (5am – 1.30pm) in the chaotic atmosphere at the community centre. There were many tired and troubled people, and she wasn't perturbed if they manifested their distress in ways which weren't accepted in her usual social circles. She didn't mind the swearing and wasn't easily deterred when arguments broke into fights. While acknowledging that using drugs and alcohol to soothe their pain was not particularly helpful, it seemed completely understandable given the circumstances. Nobody needed reminding of their mistakes. Emily felt privileged when anyone chose to confide in her, but soon discovered that allowing guests time to talk didn't always go down well with her supervisors.

## THE PROGRAMME

Almost as soon as the community centre opened, it became burdened by overcapacity; the HH board devised an interim programme to maximise assistance to men deemed most likely to successfully return to 'productive' lives. The theory behind the programme was to restore structure and a sense of purpose, alongside valuable work experience, which would be a stepping stone towards independence and future employment. Men who expressed interest in the programme were interviewed to determine their suitability. If accepted, they signed a contract agreeing to abide by a list of rules and regulations which included immediate and absolute sobriety.

Once enrolled, these men were expected to attend educational lectures and daily meetings to enhance their spiritual well-being and they were mandated to participate in 'community involvement'. Those who showed consistent commitment might later become eligible for residential placement at another facility, with more intensive rehabilitation and counselling.

The new recruits to the programme had no choice in their assignment for 'community involvement' which was also their designated work experience. They were expected to work eight-hour shifts, six days a week, and were closely monitored by case managers. For this privilege, they were allocated a permanent bed and locker in the night shelter.

A large part of Emily's job was to supervise and train the men allocated to her 'housekeeping' team for their community involvement. This was probably the least popular assignment for good reason. The housekeeping team were responsible for cleaning all of the HH facilities, including the public area within the immediate perimeter around the complex.

The men in Emily's housekeeping team had joined straight off the streets; most had already made valiant attempts to quit drugs and/or alcohol, and there was no stepped detox pathway. Absolute abstinence was expected from day one without any attempt to address the complex reasons underlying their problems. Ron, Emily's supervisor, explained that the key to their success was 'commitment to change'.

Undoubtedly the men on the programme were amazing. They kept the premises clean, the bedding laundered, and prepared food for the meals. But Emily felt uneasy, worried that they were being exploited. Her colleagues were quick to answer, "No one is forced to join the programme; they are counselled beforehand and know exactly what they're signing up for. They're free to leave at any time."

And many did leave the programme before a fortnight was up, but there always seemed to be a ready supply of replacements from amongst the hundreds who used the facility. Elise, the recently appointed director, was both sympathetic and understanding when Emily met with her and reassured her that change was on its way.

The men on the programme were mandated to attend a daily meeting run by one of the managers. Emily was seldom given the opportunity to contribute during the meetings, but when she did, it felt as though she had entered a propaganda war as she tried to shift perspectives. Emily watched all the faces in the room as she said, "Nobody wakes up one morning and decides to become addicted to drugs or alcohol, let alone end up homeless. People don't choose to lose their jobs or fall out with loved ones and end up on the street."

She desperately wanted to set the record straight that employees were there to support and not to judge. Whenever possible, Emily shared a little of her own story; it seemed to level the playing field and she hoped to provide a modicum of hope that recovery was possible, even in dire circumstances.

## CLEANING

The number of men allocated to the housekeeping team varied from day to day. They started their shift at 5.30am and the first job was to clean up outside the neighbouring businesses. There was a significant risk that the HH facilities could be shut down if they were reported as causing a public health hazard. But it was summer and makeshift tents were erected in every available space to provide shade from the heat of the day, and flimsy cover at night. It seemed futile as the housekeeping team made valiant efforts to make inroads into the filth and litter on the sidewalk around the perimeter. There were times when Emily felt as though she was mothering a group of reluctant teenagers, all in need of instruction when it came to the basic rules of hygiene. She didn't know whether to laugh or cry when she found one of her team enthusiastically using a toilet brush to scrub the hand basin in the disabled bathroom.

It was a colourful sight in the courtyard as people of all ethnicities occupied every available space, seated at the heavily graffitied square metal tables or on blankets laid on the ground. Everyone tried to make the most of the thin strips of shade beneath the overhanging roof. Extension leads covered in banks of mobile phones were plugged into the few external sockets and carefully guarded. Many people had aligned themselves to 'street families'; a reference to a sister, father, daughter etc, who was seldom a blood relative. Although there was little integration between different ethnic and racial groups, the allegiances provided a measure of stability and protection for many people who had few other allies.

## TRAINING

The Denver authorities sent out a warning about a recent outbreak of hepatitis A, amongst the homeless and Emily hoped the mandatory training on infection control would be a good forum to raise the matter of hygiene. Immunisation for the blood-borne hepatitis B virus was mandatory for client-facing staff which was wise given the number of abandoned syringes and needles, despite the sharps bins secured to the bathroom walls. Employees were assured that if they did contract a blood-borne virus, they would be covered by the 'workers' compensation scheme'. Emily was curious to know what would happen if one of the unvaccinated men on her housekeeping team were to contract hepatitis B or HIV.

It was unsettling to discover that the organisation bore no responsibility for their clients, and they advised Emily to train her team well on how to dispose of hazardous waste safely. It seemed that the homeless population were at the mercy of a system that could neither protect them nor treat them if they were to get sick as a result of their unpaid labour. Emily was reminded that participation in the programme was entirely voluntary.

Discussion of the ongoing hygiene problems was not on the agenda, even though it wasn't unusual for Emily or the housekeeping team to find themselves cleaning up human excrement and the bathrooms were in urgent need of a deep clean. Admittedly some of the people who attended the community centre were feral. Perhaps it was an act of defiance which led someone to deliberately defaecate, anywhere other than in the toilet. But it was another violation of human decency that homeless people had to endure, while they regularly encountered this sort of filth in the bathrooms earmarked for their use.

## RULE-BREAKING

Emily found it upsetting every time a member was expelled from the programme for breaching the rules. A user of crack cocaine joined the housekeeping team and begged Emily not to make him go outside to sweep the sidewalk. He was afraid of succumbing to temptation, while drug pushers continuously circled the premises. It seemed inevitable a few days later when he didn't show up for his shift and Emily couldn't reconcile how anyone could be expected to remain clean and sober without proper support. She went to see Gary, the head of the programme, who had worked at HH for years.

He listened attentively while Emily outlined why she thought it was a mistake to assign a recently clean addict to the housekeeping team. He shook his head and wagged a finger at her. "If he was really serious about staying off crack cocaine, he would do so. You need to spend more time in prayer."

Emily was stunned into silence and left his office without asking the real question, "If you were really serious about helping people get off the streets, why not at least try and reduce the chances of them succumbing to temptation? Would you ask a recovering alcoholic to work behind a bar, twenty-four hours after reaching sobriety?"

Profoundly discouraged, Emily railed against the prevailing opinion that homelessness was a direct result of 'bad' character traits, and an ethos which prescribed reform using disincentives for failure and little to motivate success. It fostered mistrust in people's basic goodness and integrity, and bore a remarkable similarity to other elitist philosophies, which perpetuate the belief that vulnerable people once 'given an inch, will take a mile'.

Thankfully, Emily's peers, the colleagues she worked with day to day, brought welcome relief with their warmth and friendship. One day, she noticed them quietly sniggering in the background. "What?" she demanded as the giggling became louder. "All I asked was whether Joe wanted to take a fag break… a cigarette," she explained, but by now they were laughing hysterically. "Oh Emily, we love your Britishness," one of her colleagues said.

They were so wholehearted in their dedication to serve others and Emily learnt a lot from them. Emily forced herself to recall what Elise had said. *Culture change is like a rudder turning around a massive tanker; it takes time to steer a big ship round.*

To survive in this job, she needed to lower her expectations and whatever she said or did required a great deal of diplomacy.

## KELLY

Around midday, Emily noticed a blonde-haired youngster with a tourniquet around her sun-tanned and lean-looking arm, sitting on the ground with a group of women. The midday sun was hot as Emily plonked herself down beside her. She whispered quietly in Kelly's ear that if she was caught, she'd be thrown out, a marker put on her card, and she'd be banned from returning to the community centre. Kelly loosened the tourniquet. Lunch was almost over but Emily managed to catch her eyes beneath the overgrown fringe and persuade her to come and get some food. While they sat together at a table in the empty dining hall, Kelly opened up:

Her mother died when she was nine years old and her father, a pastor, was left to bring her up on his own. He was never around, always off helping others from his congregation. He was ultra-strict and rarely showed affection. He beat her for trivial misdemeanours. One day, he caught her stealing money from him and counted one stroke of the cane for every cent she had taken. Kelly made up her mind to leave home as soon as she could, "to get away from him and his phoney religion." At seventeen, she joined the military, and subsequently realised she was gay. She left the army and lived with her girlfriend until they broke up. Tears streamed down Kelly's face. "I have no future – there's only thing I'm good at."

"What's that?" Emily asked.

"What I'm trained for. Killing people."

Having used cocaine occasionally, Kelly's drug habit had escalated out of control. Now she was on the streets and addicted to heroin. Kelly met up with her father once a month at a coffee shop, where he bribed her with cash, to stay away from him and his church. Kelly's features had softened during the narrative, but suddenly her demeanour changed. "See them," she said, indicating the group where she'd been sitting. "I pay them for friendship."

Kelly admitted she had to be hard; she couldn't betray her true feelings. Emily put her arm around her, moved beyond words. "How can God love me?" Kelly whispered. Emily tried to reassure her, but Kelly countered this by repeatedly saying what a failure she was and how evil it was to be a lesbian. Emily refused to agree with her. Then suddenly Kelly turned and looked Emily full in the face. With tears in her eyes she said, "You really care, don't you?"

Emily noticed the way Kelly swaggered as she walked out, apparently full of confidence. Colleagues had warned her about Kelly. She had a reputation for violence, but Emily had seen someone else – a young girl, rejected by her religious father who had failed to give her the love and comfort every child deserves. Like many who frequented the community centre, Kelly disappeared off the scene and Emily was left wondering what had happened to her.

## NOT A HERO

It was obvious that many guests used aggression as a survival strategy which had nothing to do with their true nature. Rather it was a reflection of the horrors they had endured and the never-ending nightmares that still plagued their lives. Although Emily felt genuinely touched by the affirmation of guests, she knew she was no superhero. A normal day was enough to bring Emily rapidly down to earth. Often, after the doors opened at 5.30am, she had no break, no chance to drink or pee and left her shift an hour late, stressed, and exhausted. She witnessed assaults, dealt with reports of theft amongst those who had few belongings. She was frequently subjected to verbal abuse. She didn't always respond with grace and was perfectly capable of getting angry, frustrated, or irritated just like anyone else.

Although Emily's work distracted her from her own troubles and gave her more perspective, she didn't deny that she was still recovering herself, and as she told everyone else, "There is no league table of pain." But somewhat surprisingly, work gave her valuable mental space, enough to prioritise what was important and she continued her counselling with Barb.

\* \* \*

*Are you someone who feels that your problems are unjustified compared to the difficulties other people face? Perhaps being kind to yourself and giving yourself permission to have needs, may be an important step towards recovery.*

# CHAPTER 31

# Assault

Emily had severe tennis elbow. Her medical insurance wouldn't cover work-related problems and so she found herself consulting the workers' compensation doctor. Dr Jay issued strict instructions that Emily was not to lift anything or perform any further manual cleaning tasks at work, so on the day when no one from the housekeeping roster turned up for their shift, Emily needed help. But Tim, her new supervisor, was not available.

## SOLO

The sidewalk around the facility perimeter looked like a slum; every available space between the street tents was covered in litter and discarded bits of food. Many people were still asleep on makeshift mattresses. Emily's priority had to be to clear up outside the nearby business premises, at least to avoid their inevitable complaints. Emily tried to sweep up and then empty the trash cans but as she pushed the wheelie bin along, it caught on a paving stone and toppled over. Thankfully, a couple of guys came to the rescue, but they melted away just as soon as they had uprighted it for her. She trundled the full wheelie bin down the alleyway to empty it in the dumpster, some way beyond the facility. The alleyway smelt like a latrine, and she passed several piles of faeces and bits of used toilet paper. She stopped when she saw the crack-cocaine addict who had gone AWOL and crouched down beside him, trying to ignore the pile of poo beside her. He told her how he had found some crack behind a trash can... and afterwards he had felt too ashamed, couldn't face anyone. He was obviously in a bad way, dirty, dishevelled, sleeping on the street. He elaborated further on his misery – how he'd been brought up as a Christian and how he'd let God down. Emily couldn't persuade him otherwise, nor could she coax him inside, even for something to eat. He didn't raise his eyes as he shook his head. "It's no use, I've been here before. I can't change!"

Unable to do any more, Emily left him and carried on down the alleyway pulling the wheelie bin behind her. Another man approached and started shouting; he closed in on her as Emily retreated, only to find herself pinned against the wall. With his face in hers, he ranted and raved, angry because she had stopped his girlfriend from bringing her cat into the community centre.

Emily recalled the incident. Animals were not allowed on HH premises, and this woman had been aggressive, insisting that the poor cat, locked in a filthy plastic box, was a service animal. Emily had referred the decision to her supervisor, but Tim was adamant. "No way is any animal allowed in, especially under false pretences."

Now virtually alone in the alleyway with her aggressor, Emily shouted back as loudly as she could, "I did not make the rules. If you're unhappy, go see my boss."

Surprisingly he backed off and trembling, Emily carried on to the dumpster without looking back. On her hurried return, the addict still held his head in his hands, certainly in no fit state to rescue her. She had been lucky.

There was a message that Gary wanted to see her. Emily knocked on his door and was invited into his homely office and ushered to a comfortable chair. He said he'd heard that she was upset. After Emily outlined the morning's problems, with a smile on his face, he asked whether she'd spent time in prayer before coming to work. Emily answered, "Right now, prayer is the last thing on my mind. I need help to get the priority jobs done."

"Emily, Emily," he replied, "Jesus will give you grace enough to see you through the day."

She left his office speechless with fury. *Was Jesus going to help clean the streets or empty the overflowing trash cans? Was Jesus going to pick up the litter around the shop doorways or answer the business owners' complaints when they called with demands to come and clear up 'your' people's mess? Would Jesus don PPE to clear the hazardous waste, like the faeces in the alleyway?* Finally, her inner rant gave way to tears, and she worried who would replenish the toilet paper and soap, let alone clean the dormitories.

## PERSECUTION

One of the men who usually worked on the late shift came to help as Emily cleaned up dog poop which was all down the ramp leading to the community centre entrance. She listened while he described how one of the sidewalk campers had come over, snatched the dustpan from his hand and thrown it across the street, hurling abuse at him. It had taken every fibre of his being to stop himself from hitting the guy. The men who helped on the housekeeping team were easy targets for other people's frustrations. Another time, Emily had planted herself between her team member, Tony, and another man on the street, to stop a fight. Tony had laughed. "Emily, you don't need to protect me."

He was right, it was ridiculous. Nevertheless, it felt unbearable to see him dragged into trouble. He'd been sober for weeks, determined to save up until he could afford to travel back to his family in another state and the chance of a fresh start.

## SURPRISE

It was September and nothing seemed unusual when one of the women asked for Emily's help. The only shower available for women was strictly timetabled. If not adhered to, tempers amongst the waiting women became frayed. At the five-minute warning, there had been no response and so Emily was summoned. She had reason to feel anxious, having already found one woman unconscious from an overdose of heroin. When her shout and knocking was met with silence, Emily unlocked and tentatively opened the door, but there was no sign of the woman. Then suddenly there was a loud bang, and everyone was screaming. Emily's glasses were on the floor, and she heard colleagues asking if she was all right. The woman must have been behind the door and slammed it shut, catching Emily's head in the door-frame.

She was in the office where colleagues were urgently discussing what to do next; they decided this woman must be barred from the premises and her HH ID card revoked.

When the woman finally emerged from the bathroom, her head covered with a hoodie, she walked slowly, defiantly over to the office. All Emily remembers is her asking for the ID card. Emily didn't feel any pain, but the world had taken on a strange quality as though she was viewing it from a distance. Apparently, she had been assaulted a second time.

By the time the police arrived, the woman was long gone. Emily declined the offer of an ambulance but one of her colleagues drove her to the medical centre to see Dr Jay. Still unable to remember what had happened, Emily's jaw ached, her arm hurt and she felt nauseous and exhausted. The doctor checked her over and was happy that she hadn't sustained any significant injury.

It wasn't until Emily was in the shower at home, that she realised her hair was matted with blood, her head was swollen, and the wound was still bleeding. Even when she returned to the medical centre, she still had no recollection of the attack. Dr Jay examined her again and asked the nurses to clean and glue the two wounds on her head.

Tim seemed annoyed when she rang to ask if she could come in late the next day. It was the homeless people who expressed surprise that she was back at work at all. Several of them offered to 'watch her back'. As it happened, Emily found herself supervising one of the well-known addicts who was high. Having managed to get him seated for some breakfast, she was astonished to see her assailant calmly eating at a table nearby.

The woman had obviously managed to get in, even without her ID card. Emily requested assistance on her two-way radio, but she slipped away a second time. The police asked Emily to press charges; apparently this was necessary before they could issue a warrant for her arrest. Having identified that this was not her first violent assault, Emily hoped that at least she might get some help before anything worse happened.

## ANXIETY

It was good to be off at the weekend and Emily made light of the attack. But at her next session, Barb was not impressed by Emily's nonchalance as she described it as an occupational hazard. "Emily, this is serious. It is not okay. Nobody has checked up on you or offered support. You should have been ushered away from the area immediately after the first attack and you should not have returned to work so soon."

Suddenly Emily's bravado crumpled, and she admitted she felt anxious and unsafe at work, knowing that her unpredictable assailant was still at large. Barb insisted that she return to see Dr Jay. They were about to take their first trip back to England and Dr Jay signed Emily off work; she would review the situation once Emily returned from her holiday.

Changes were afoot, Tim left HH without giving notice and then Gary left too and Emily was emailed by another new supervisor: *When are you coming back to work?*

It didn't make sense that Emily still felt so anxious; it was as though her brain had been reset to 'high alert' and she kept looking around as though an attack might come from any direction. It never occurred to her that these symptoms may also have been compounded as a result of withdrawal from venlafaxine.

Jeremy, one of Emily's colleagues, urgently needed a place to stay and moved into their spare room the day they arrived back from England. After a couple of weeks, he confirmed that management were not overly sympathetic about the assault. Without proper support, Emily felt unable to return to work and so she offered her resignation.

She made a brief visit to HH to say goodbye and it was the homeless people who gathered round and enquired after her health. One of the more notorious men nicknamed 'Goldfinger' patted her on the shoulder. They hadn't always seen eye to eye, but now he said he was sorry about what happened. Another said he was glad she wasn't coming back only because he didn't want HH to break her. Emily knew she would genuinely miss these wonderful people who had already survived so much adversity and had so little hope that their circumstances would change.

## WORKERS' COMP

Emily's battle with anxiety continued and she constantly felt on edge. They had always said their lives were never boring, but at this point boring sounded attractive. Her usual health insurance would not provide cover since the assault was classified as a 'work-related injury'. Even though Emily no longer worked at HH, she was still obliged to receive her medical care for the assault and her tennis elbow, through the workers' compensation scheme. But she discovered that her medical bills were only covered if she demonstrated full compliance with the advice of their doctors. It meant Emily was obliged to attend every appointment and this in turn, generated a report which was also copied to her ex-employer.

It had been puzzling when a neighbour advised her to hire a lawyer and it would have saved her a whole load of stress if she had done so from the start; she needed help to negotiate through the complexities of the workers' compensation scheme.

Dr Jay had diagnosed an 'acute stress reaction' as a direct result of the assault and advised psychotherapy. Thankfully, she approved Barb as the therapist because Emily could no longer afford to see her, and the scheme agreed to pay the bill.

It was a surprise to discover that she was also entitled to some financial relief because her resignation was directly related to the assault. But Emily also discovered that she was not allowed to apply for any other jobs until the scheme deemed her fit to do so. It was exceptionally difficult when this vital source of income was erroneously terminated on several occasions without notice. The battle to get the weekly payments reinstated was hardly conducive to recovery.

## INJUNCTION

There was a phone call from the state prosecutor's office to inform Emily of her assailant's arrest and the issue of an injunction which prohibited her from being within a one-hundred-foot radius. Emily was instructed to carry this document on her person at all times and call 911 if it was violated. But when the injunction arrived in the post, it was made out to someone else and did nothing to allay Emily's fears that the assailant now knew her address. In late December, the state prosecutor called again. During the second court appearance, her assailant had started to scream and shout, so the judge sent her for a four-week psychiatric evaluation. It was some comfort to know that she would be receiving medical attention.

## FREEZE

At Christmas, Emily invited some of her homeless friends for lunch. She drove down to HH on a snowy day and while she sat waiting in the car, someone knocked on the window. Startled, Emily went into a state of complete panic, frozen with fear, unable to move. The man was persistent, insisting that she come inside to the warmth, and eventually with heart still racing, Emily managed to struggle out of the car. Once inside, she smiled and nodded as people greeted her, but it was as if they were speaking a foreign language, as she fought against the terror which threatened to overwhelm her.

Despite the freezing temperatures outside, the January sun felt warm through the window. Emily sat at her desk in the bedroom, staring up at the blue sky and wondering what 2018 would bring. Although the sessions with Barb were helpful, the debilitating episodes of anxiety had become more frequent. They weren't anything like the classic panic attacks she knew from her medical training. Suddenly she'd be struck with an overwhelming desire to flee, as though from some great danger. On a couple of occasions, she had actually taken off without any idea where she was going; it was embarrassing, illogical and difficult to explain.

# DEVELOPMENTS

Barb suggested that Emily sign up for an 'inner-healing' session and despite her scepticism Emily thought there was nothing to lose. Barb also wrote to Dr Jay asking for another review. Dr Jay ordered an MRI scan of her brain and also referred her to the workers' compensation scheme psychiatrist. Emily was mortified by the idea of a psychiatric assessment. She also thought the scan was pointless three months after the assault, but had no choice, when failure to cooperate might stop all her financial support and land her with all the medical bills to boot.

Emily met with the three members of the prayer team at the church; they asked her some very personal and searching questions and she answered as honestly as she could. Then she was asked to systematically verbalise forgiveness towards everyone she could think of past and present who could have possibly hurt her. Emily found the exercise surprisingly cathartic.

It was a relief to receive confirmation that the workers' compensation scheme had accepted liability, which meant they agreed to pay all her medical bills. But she was still mandated to attend the scheduled psychiatry appointments.

The MRI report was slightly disturbing. Although there were no 'gross changes', the scan showed minor abnormalities which could be 'as a result of past trauma'. Dr Jay didn't know if this was significant or not. Emily was worried that these findings were sequelae from the head injury and it didn't occur to her that they could possibly evidence damage resulting from the multiple episodes of ECT she had had in the past.

She emailed Professor Scott in Dundee to try and retrieve her post-surgery MRI scans for comparison. They had continued to exchange emails occasionally, and Emily had thought she had been tactful when she reported how Barb had different views about her diagnosis of depression. Professor Scott was usually very prompt with his replies, so when she didn't hear back, she hoped it was because he was busy rather than offended.

When the state prosecutor's office rang for the third time, it was to inform Emily that her assailant had been released after her psychiatric evaluation. Apparently, she had been found 'unfit to stand trial by reason of insanity' and returned to the streets because the state had insufficient resources to offer either treatment or housing. Emily was terrified.

## AMERICAN SHRINK

The appointment with the psychiatrist was completely different from anything she had experienced in the UK. His 'office' was located in a row of fairly small and non-descript terraced houses in a residential area. There was no doorbell and finding the front door unlocked, Emily walked straight into a small room. It was completely empty except for a few comfortable chairs and some magazines, and she sat herself down wondering if she was in the right place. When she heard voices coming through the wall, loud enough to hear what was being said, it was obvious a consultation was in progress. The lack of privacy was unnerving to say the least. Fighting her instinct to run away, Emily waited.

After ten minutes or so, the client/patient left through the front door, and the psychiatrist ushered Emily into a room that looked like a cross between a personal study and a sitting room. He seemed relaxed as he plied Emily with questions although he didn't appear to be paying much attention to the answers.

He agreed with Dr Jay, that she was suffering from an acute stress reaction, and advised Emily to continue the psychotherapy. But he also suggested she needed drug treatment as he got up out of his chair to pull out a large plastic box from a shelf on the bookcase. He rooted around inside and handed Emily some free samples of duloxetine. Emily tried to counter this by telling him she had previously suffered severe adverse effects. "Just give it a try," he said as he also wrote a prescription for an increased dose of trazodone and a benzodiazepine which he wanted her to take regularly to control the episodes of panic.

When she got back home, Emily consigned the duloxetine samples to the bin but filled the prescriptions for the other medication at Walgreens, just in case anyone checked.

A month later, Emily had a second appointment and explained that she couldn't tolerate the duloxetine because of what she had been through on venlafaxine. He didn't seem unduly concerned but was very insistent that she should take a regular dose of clonazepam instead. He seemed puzzled by Emily's reluctance. She explained her medical background and her concerns that benzodiazepines were addictive. He replied, "Is that a problem?"

Undoubtedly stress can push inner resources to the limit, and it was lucky that Emily was sufficiently disenchanted with psychiatric drugs to be able to resist having them reinstated. It was also fortunate that Barb was not wedded to the idea of medication. Despite her religious bias, she helped Emily understand that her symptoms were not primarily a medical problem and with a little more time, she would soon be back to normal.

* * *

*What resources do you need to believe that recovery is possible? Even when bad things happen, with the right support, maybe you can find the hope you need.*

# CHAPTER 32

# Resolution

Peter's job had come to an end but like Emily, he was simultaneously underqualified and overexperienced. He could practise as a Colorado *registered* psychotherapist, but he could not become *licensed* without an American postgraduate degree, which was very restrictive.

## DISCOVERIES

It became apparent why their neighbour had been so insistent that Emily would need an attorney. Her case could only be closed after a judge determined the amount of the settlement which would pay Emily's medical bills accrued since the injuries. An estimate for any future medical care must also be considered because the usual health insurance would not cover any long-term sequelae following a work-related injury. It was a considerable strain and added greatly to the existing financial pressure the couple were under.

The days were lengthening, and they looked forward to lighter evenings. One weekend, Emily spotted an advertisement for a dance class in the local paper. The class was already underway when Emily opened the door into the hall at the community centre. Women of various ages and abilities were clearly enjoying themselves as they went through a prolonged warm-up routine set to well-known pop songs. Tentatively she joined in at the back of the hall, and at a break Emily introduced herself to the teachers, Nora, and Hannah. She hadn't done any kind of dance for many years, but she soon made friends with the class participants and 'Encore Dance' became a wonderful distraction. It was impossible to think about her problems while learning the steps for an upcoming performance.

Through the dance class connections, Emily was introduced to the amateur dramatics group, which also took place in the community centre. Peter also became involved, and it opened doors to new friendships. When Emily joined the Aurora Writers' Group, she found a new lease of life as she started writing fiction; some of the skits she wrote were later performed by the drama group.

Nevertheless, she was not completely out of the woods; one day she was driving a familiar route to a writers' meeting, when for no apparent reason, the panic hit. She pulled over to the side of the road, where she sat clutching the steering wheel, as she tried to get a grip on herself, turn the car round and drive home. It felt as though she was walking across a meadow, blissfully unaware of trip-wires hidden in the grass until suddenly she found herself flat on her face.

Peggy, one of Emily's author friends, told her the story of her family's escape from the Mormon church. It was shocking to hear the outrageous abasement they had gone through, and yet Peggy still battled with her conscience, tormented by the guilt of seemingly abandoning God. This provoked Emily to re-examine her own church experience and it seemed like another epiphany when Emily realised her own susceptibility to control and coercion, which she had witnessed or experienced in so many settings throughout her life. It really was time to break free.

## COURT

In June 2018, the attorney accompanied Peter and Emily to the pre-settlement court hearing for the closure of Emily's case with the workers' compensation scheme. The judge awarded Emily the maximum compensation allowed for pain and suffering which is low in these cases, circa one thousand dollars, and also a sum towards future care. The medical bills were paid, the lawyer took his agreed percentage, and there was not much left, other than relief that it was finally over.

Even Barb recognised and respected how Emily was becoming less engaged with the fundamentalist Christian views of their church. She suggested House for All Sinners and Saints (HFASS). Neither Peter nor Emily had heard of the minister and founder, Nadia Bolz-Weber who was famous as the author of two *NY Times* bestselling books. They visited HFASS purely out of curiosity, and it also happened to be the day Nadia announced she was handing over her role to her assistant pastor, Jack. It was refreshing to find out that he was openly gay, living with his partner and a substantial proportion of the congregation identified as LGBTQ+. The sermons were short, poignant, filled with more wisdom in ten minutes than they had heard in years. But Emily felt as though her faith was unravelling and her previous beliefs about Christianity fell apart at the seams.

She did, however, decide to keep going to the services at HFASS. At least there she felt free to confront her doubts and ask difficult questions. The people she met seemed both authentic and accepting and everyone was welcomed regardless of their beliefs, background, or circumstances.

It felt as if scales had fallen from her eyes, and slowly Emily began to feel a renewed sense of peace through a very different expression of the Christian faith, neither tied to evangelicalism nor the charismatic church. On many levels it felt like a metamorphosis, as all that Emily had previously believed to be true about her life and experience was undergoing profound change.

## FOOT SURGERY

In October 2018, Emily was due to have major surgery on her foot and planned to use the opportunity to completely stop the trazodone; she would be sleepy from the anaesthetic and would also benefit from the sedating properties of the painkillers.

A few days after the operation, Emily started to experience some very strange symptoms: first, her foot went completely numb and she was worried the plaster was too tight, but it was checked, and they advised Emily not to elevate the leg too high. The sensation returned as very painful pins and needles, which shortly developed into an extreme burning sensation. Unable to sleep, the only relief Emily could find was outside in the freezing air of the balcony. The following day Emily returned to the medical centre and insisted they remove the plaster. They tried to put her in a splint, but she couldn't bear anything touching her foot.

The orthopaedic surgeon diagnosed a peripheral neuropathy but insisted it was completely unrelated to the surgery. He prescribed gabapentin to treat nerve pain alongside a lignocaine cream which was a local anaesthetic. He also reassured her that it was unlikely to be a long-term problem. The extreme pain began to subside, but nothing seemed to relieve the symptoms completely.

Emily cannot be sure when she became aware that her other foot was also affected, nor did she connect the fact that her symptoms arose almost directly after suddenly stopping trazodone. The burning pain worsened in the evenings and when her feet were warm, disturbing sleep – and the symptoms persist to this day. Eventually, Emily was diagnosed with small fibre neuropathy.

Years later, I found out more about protracted withdrawal syndrome from antidepressants, which is far more likely to occur when psychiatric drugs like trazodone are stopped suddenly or tapered too fast. Other people have reported similar symptoms after stopping antidepressants and although I cannot be sure, it seems likely that stopping trazodone precipitously may have caused the problem.

## OFF MEDICATION

Without this knowledge and despite the symptoms, Emily celebrated the fact that she was finally off all the antidepressants that she had been taking for the last fifteen years. She had been experiencing periods of intense emotion even before she had completely stopped venlafaxine, but reassured herself that she was making up for lost time when she found herself crying far more readily than she was used to. Emily didn't see this release of emotion as a bad thing, on the contrary, she saw it as healing. What a contrast it was to the past, when it would have worried her a great deal, wondering if it was a sign of relapse.

Now Emily knew for certain that for years her emotions had been numbed by antidepressants, but now she was no longer afraid of her true emotional self. Perhaps the panic and anxiety associated with the assault may also have been an exaggerated emotional response as part of a withdrawal reaction; it had coincided exactly with the time when Emily had stopped venlafaxine.

Even though Emily admitted to experiencing painful and extreme emotions at times, she also felt liberated and revelled in her new-found ability to laugh and feel intense joy. Her sleep remained disturbed but still she congratulated herself that she had made it through all the stress and anxiety of the last few years without recourse to long-term psychiatric drugs. Emily felt more emotionally healthy than she had ever been before.

## MEDIA REPORTS

During the autumn of 2018 the American news was full of the Ford versus Kavanaugh hearings. Christine Blasey Ford's allegations of sexual assault by Brett Kavanaugh, one of Trump's nominees for a position on the supreme court, had become public knowledge. Ford had been a teenager at the time of the alleged assault, and this had led to heated debate around the subject of sexual violence towards women and girls.

At one of the Sunday services, Jack, the pastor at HFASS, very sensitively voiced his suspicion that some people in the congregation may be triggered by the recent media storm. He handled it beautifully as he offered support to anyone who had been sexually abused or betrayed. Emily was surprised at how emotional she had been during the service and afterwards, Jack came over to check if she was all right. It was slightly embarrassing since Emily hadn't personally been subjected to any kind of sexual assault in the past.

It was serendipity when later that week, one of Emily's friends from England called and during their long catch-up chat, Emily explained how she was feeling. Emily was amazed when her friend disclosed her own experience of abuse at the hands of an influential church leader. While Emily mulled over the latest revelation, her anger boiled over. Emily looked back to the time when she was a vulnerable teenager, now convinced of the suspicion that she had never revealed to anyone. There was a connection between the two men and suddenly Emily was certain that Jasper had knowingly orchestrated the compromising and sexually risky position he had put her in at age fourteen.

The despicable betrayal by male predators who also happened to be highly regarded within church circles made Emily wonder how many young people suffered silently at their hands. What hypocrites these men were. How could they live with themselves? What horrors children the world over have been subjected to, whether sexual violence or other forms of abuse, at the hands of those entrusted with their care. Yet few of these children will ever get justice.

## CONFRONTING CHANGE

Despite Emily's growing cynicism towards Christianity, at least she still felt comfortable to be associated with HFASS, where discussion about difficult subjects such as sexual abuse was not avoided. In this community, people were accepted whatever their past or present struggles. It felt like a sanctuary filled with love, compassion, and empathy. It was refreshing to come across a church which was not obsessed by the desire to fix people or 'heal' them with prayer.

Even though Peter and Emily felt settled and happy in their Denver home, they still desperately needed to earn a living. Emily doubled her efforts to find work and took a course in journalism. Sheila, from the 'Federation of Women in Business', had high hopes that Emily could make a career by writing and speaking. She offered to help her apply for grants and advertise her services. But everything Emily put her hand to required further financial investment. Together, Peter and Emily were forced to face the seriousness of their situation. As immigrants, they had to be resident in the country for seven years before they would be entitled to any help and the risk that future healthcare might become unaffordable was too much. Reluctantly they decided to return to the UK.

There was just one thing left to do before leaving Denver. Emily had her arms tattooed. Perhaps the blue-black images of flowers would distract people's attention away from what was very evidently underneath. This time when she returned to work in A&E, she hoped her new colleagues might get to know her first before they noticed the scars.

In 2019, before they left for England, Emily met pastor Jack for coffee. He listened while she described how their emigration to Denver had turned into an unmitigated disaster and how deluded she had been in thinking that they were doing the right thing. She admitted she felt resentful at being forced to leave Denver just when they had finally found happiness. It had all turned out to be a rather expensive nightmare of a 'vacation' which had cost them their life savings. She told Jack that when they arrived she thought she was following God, but now she was leaving, she wasn't even sure God existed. He simply looked at Emily with his clear blue eyes and simply asked, "How do you know that this was not God's plan for you?"

For some people, loss of 'faith' can be deeply disturbing and may manifest in ways which can be misinterpreted as mental illness. Although Emily was experiencing an existential faith crisis, given time to reflect, she realised that disappointments and failures in life are rarely wholly bad and may be used as a time of personal growth. She realised that for her, she could continue to benefit her mental health through writing, dance, and drama.

\* \* \*

*We should not underestimate the value of artistic expression, music, movement, creativity, or that of spirituality, all of which can be catalysts to recovery, and a focus for our well-being. Are there people or activities which might help you to reconnect with life in a different way? It may be a matter of trial and error to find what is right for you.*

# CHAPTER 33

# Return to England

## MY VOICE

The gradual emergence of who I am today, someone who feels much more integrated and recovered from serious mental illness, has been ongoing. When we arrived back in the UK, I was a very different person to the one who had left to emigrate to America.

I didn't want to leave Denver and I didn't want to return to medicine again. I didn't enjoy the flight back to England, but I couldn't help feeling better as we travelled by train from Gatwick. The lush, green countryside of the English spring in 2019 raised my spirits and I looked forward to catching up with the rest of our family.

We were moving to temporary accommodation in an area where we hadn't lived before, and I didn't underestimate how stressful the settling in period would be. We needed to sell the apartment and had left most of our belongings behind. Peter was also looking for work.

Given the current stresses, plus the added combination of

shift work in my new job in A&E, and the ongoing pain from the neuropathy, it was hardly surprising that I wasn't sleeping well. I continued to be proactive in managing my mental health and made an appointment with a professional therapist who specialised in counselling doctors. I explained why I wanted to talk to someone independent who understood the stress of returning to medicine after two and a half years away, and would listen without resorting to panic, given my previous psychiatric history. Stress and anxiety seemed a very reasonable reaction to our current situation and the therapist agreed. By the time of the second appointment, I was already feeling much better.

Before leaving Denver I had discovered that the neurosurgeon who performed Emily's operation had been struck off the medical register in the UK. I contacted the Advanced Interventions Service in Dundee, and was quickly reassured on the phone, that none of his alleged surgical misdemeanours involved the patients on the NMD research programme. Nonetheless, it was extremely disconcerting. The experimental surgery I underwent is no longer practised in Dundee, although the AIS continue to send patients for certain interventions to Queen's Hospital for neurosurgery in London.

## EPIPHANY

I didn't set out to change my opinions. I didn't set out to change my views about psychiatry even when I started reducing my medication. It never occurred to me that what I learned from Peter as he trained to become a counsellor, or paying to see an American psychotherapist would dramatically change my outlook. My complete U-turn in thinking was never an act of rebellion, nor was it without cost to me personally. However, I have been fortunate to get support to tackle so many of the painful problems which had been running along in the background throughout my adult life, although I believe the healing process will continue for the rest of my days. I think I was also very lucky to not have had worse reactions when I withdrew from medication. Many others do not fare so well.

But up until 2019, I still felt out on a limb in the medical world. I did not know of any other doctors, particularly psychiatrists, who would validate what I now believed about my past. It was quite fortuitous that I came across an article by the Child and Adolescent Psychiatrist, Dr Sami Timimi. I wrote to him and as a result, was introduced to the Critical Psychiatry Network.

This group is made up mainly of psychiatrists, many of whom are consultants and work in the UK. Here was a group of professionals who openly expressed their doubts over the validity of psychiatric diagnosis and/or have scrutinised the research and evidence to support the use of psychotropic drugs and ECT. I have found the network both stimulating and enlightening and even though opinions may differ over what constitutes optimal treatment, they universally believe in accountability and transparency.

As I continued to read more about the history of psychiatry and found websites such as Mad in America and the International Institute for Psychiatric Drug Withdrawal, I was both heartened and dismayed to find that I am amongst many survivors who share similar experiences. I read Bessel van der Kolk's book, *The Body Keeps the Score* and Johann Hari's *Lost Connections: why you're depressed and how to find hope,* amongst others. There are many contributions both from professionals and from survivors, all of whom hold alternative views to traditional biomedical psychiatry as practised in the West. It increasingly felt as though we'd been duped when it came to psychiatric diagnoses and treatments. I discovered that the research which I had always assumed underpinned the central tenets of psychiatry was full of ambiguities. There was no concrete evidence for any of the treatment I had endured. Like so many patients and doctors alike, I had listened without question to the myths about 'depression' – like the serotonin theory, presented in scientific language and widely peddled as fact. Yet the truth that there was no evidence of chemical imbalance and no evidence of structural or genetic brain defects, had remained well hidden beneath the respectability of the medical discipline known as psychiatry.

It has been sobering to conclude that all those years ago when I worked at the Royal Cornhill Hospital, I had been right to question how patients received their diagnoses. Diagnostic labels are nothing more than opinionated descriptions made by psychiatrists, in an attempt to categorise patients' difficulties, and give them treatment, usually with psychiatric drugs. Yet there is still no scientific basis for psychiatric diagnosis, nor justification for many of the treatments which are so widely advocated for patients who consult their doctors with psychological or emotional problems.

## ENLIGHTENED

With the benefit of hindsight, I can see just how easy it is to be dominated and influenced by so-called expertise. It took years for me to discover that the medication I was prescribed was never going to make my depressive symptoms go away or stay away. I endured so much hardship while drugged to the eyeballs and suffering from side effects. What I experienced was transcribed in my medical record, written as medical jargon, for example– 'psychomotor retardation' – the layman would say 'slowed' up. The fact that I was over-sedated as a result of the medication and that my memory was shot to pieces by the ECT was not taken into consideration. It seems obvious that I would be unable to make progress in psychotherapy given such circumstances. I was coerced on numerous occasions, incarcerated on locked psychiatric wards, then later grateful to my captors for my release.

Over twenty years later and my rational mind informs me that no one from that period has the power to hurt me anymore. Yet my body has still not completely recovered and occasionally I still feel the dry mouth, the tightening of my muscles and the sensation of my heart racing in the vicinity of the places where I was hospitalised.

## UNCERTAINTIES

I don't know if the same psychiatrists who were involved in my care continue to hold to their original views. It is possible that they will continue to defend the position they took then. Maybe they will say that I was extremely ill and incapable of making valid decisions for myself; that I needed to be sectioned, detained in hospital against my will and forced to take medication and given ECT, in my best interests. Very likely they will say that most of the time I gave my full consent to treatment.

Yet I did not know that my diagnosis lacked validity. I did not know that the evidence for the effectiveness of ECT is lacking, even though I came to understand that it was damaging to my memory. I did not know there was no evidence that the drugs they prescribed would ever make me better. I was not prepared for the adverse effects. It was only relatively recently that I discovered that the burning in my feet from 'small fibre neuropathy' and the persistent insomnia are very likely part of a protracted withdrawal syndrome. I was not warned that this was a possibility.

Maybe the psychiatrists didn't know these things either, but now there is no excuse. Patients must be made aware of all the options. There must be candid discussions and transparency. Drug companies and others have contrived to make false claims over the efficacy of many psychiatric drugs and have denied their harms. This deception must stop.

While I came to terms with just how little my psychiatrists

really knew about what caused my distress that they diagnosed as depression, or the treatments they prescribed, I felt angry. Despite this, my admiration for those who work in mental health services and to the best of their ability, try to help their very disturbed and distressed patients, has not diminished. Nonetheless, I believe it was through psychiatry's ignorance that I suffered needlessly. It was damaging to me as an individual and as a consequence, it indirectly hurt my family. While it is easy to fall into the trap of believing that the mistakes resulted from the personal failures of certain individuals, this is not the case. Rather they are pawns within our culture and political system that allows traditional psychiatric practice to continue.

* * *

*Are you aware of your options? Have you had all the information you need to make decisions about any interventions offered or any drugs prescribed? Are you able to have candid conversations with the professionals who are responsible for providing your care? It is important to be fully informed before giving your consent and that means having all the questions that you want to ask, answered to your satisfaction.*

# CHAPTER 34

# Deeper healing

Undoubtedly Barb had been helpful, but I was aware that Christian beliefs had saddled me with some deep-seated and unhelpful narratives. I wondered how I had remained wedded to evangelicalism for so long. I felt ashamed that I had been deceived by the psychiatric paradigm and undergone years of unnecessary treatment which robbed my children of a normal family life.

## GINA

It was good to meet Gina, who helped me process and reframe more of my experiences. She encouraged me to accept myself for who I am and what I had been through. With her help I was able to accept that I have always been a worthwhile person and reject the religious premise instilled in me that I was born bad.

Gina also recognised how damaging the boarding school experience had been; it was the big chestnut. Even Barb hadn't guessed its size and I embarked on a further journey of healing which could so easily have taken place decades earlier. Then the pandemic hit, and our sessions had to stop. During lockdown, I read and researched more on the problems faced by ex-boarders. I remain curious why, over the many years I spent as a psychiatric patient, so little attention was paid to my frequent references of the torment I faced as a child.

## BOARDING SCHOOL SYNDROME

Several books have had a big impact on me. The first of which was *Boarding School Syndrome: The psychological trauma of the privileged child* by Joy Schaverien. I was bowled over by the discovery that so many others had also suffered a great deal during later life as a result of their boarding school years and why so little attention has been given to us.

Children sent away to school at younger ages, appear to be more susceptible and Schaverien describes what I so succinctly remember – the mismatch between the overly positive message given by the parents and the reality of the child's lived experience. Now it seems so obvious how damaging it is to a young child just by the way it tears them in two. No wonder so many boarders developed similar coping strategies to deal with their distress, and are later prone to similar patterns of problems, manifesting as addictions, severe relationship problems, and symptoms which may lead to psychiatric diagnoses. Schaverien describes both the complexities and the hiddenness of the long-term effects. Sadly, when these are unrecognised some ex-boarders may even succumb to suicide. She describes how many ex-boarders still cannot face talking about their experiences even decades later.

I was interested in another less obvious phenomenon whereby some ex-boarders become overly dependent on 'success'. The latter group appear to do well in life, get to the top and are very intolerant of others who they perceive to be showing weakness, simply because they cannot allow their own feelings out of the box... this can lead to callous and bullying behaviour which then propagates the problem for future generations. I could certainly identify with this theory which is also well described by both Nick Duffell in his book, *The Making of Them: The British Attitude to Children and the Boarding School System* and Richard Beard's *Sad Little Men: Private Schools and the Ruin of England*. In the latter, I was particularly struck by his description of the wall of silence that has epitomised the worst of the western ideologies where we would rather bury our mistakes than own them.

In my own life, I had perfected the ability to turn uncomfortable feelings into hard work and became accustomed to silencing my emotions. To the uninitiated outsider, especially to an employer, this may seem very healthy, laudable even. But it is not sustainable and, in my life, burn-out preceded the inevitable collapse.

As I reflected on the fact that numerous references exist describing the misery young children suffer when abandoned at residential schools, either in novels, or in biographies, it felt even more puzzling that I hadn't been listened to during the years of psychiatric treatment.

It was as early as 1990, that Nick Duffell first brought the problems faced by adult boarding school survivors to the attention of the national press along with the concept that boarding school could be very damaging to children. In 1994, his BBC documentary *The Making of Them*, shed further light on the plight of the privileged child sent away from home at a young age. *It was later that same year, that Emily was diagnosed with depression and first came to the attention of psychiatry.* Nick Duffell's sentinel book of the same name was published in 2000, a coherent account of how children survive under such circumstances. It was reviewed in the *BMJ. This also failed to ring any bells to those who were caring for Emily's mental health.* In retrospect, I wish that my therapists and psychiatrists had read this book. Surely it would have changed their perspectives.

It was also helpful to discover the differences between the single sex boarding schools. In boys' schools, reports of abuse are predominantly physical, whereas in girls' schools, control is maintained by coercion. Emotional neglect was ubiquitous in all schools, *but the harm done to girls has been grossly underestimated when there was neither a physical, nor a sexual element to the abuse.* It was enlightening to learn from the collated experience of others and therefore to understand more fully how Emily came to display certain characteristics or traits, in later life.

Those who work with ex-boarders confirm the universality of how children develop an appearance of coping and superficial happiness while at boarding school. Of course, there are some children who appear to have suffered no ill effects at all and as adults appear very happy with their boarding school education. Yet it cannot be right that hundreds, even thousands of ex-boarders are now disclosing how lost, confused and utterly miserable they felt at school and how the effects have continued to plague them in their adult lives.

Since then, I have had the opportunity to talk to many ex-boarders, including some old school friends; many had made similar interpretations of their experiences. There are many tragic stories, and I heard many others describe years of misery at school. Yet all of us felt isolated, unaware that we were not alone in our suffering. This same sense of isolation continued into our adult lives, and for some it is only very recently that they have met other ex-boarders and have started the journey to healing. One friend described the reunion at their former school as 'confronting the demons'.

## OPENING UP TO TRUTH

I have had to own up to my blindness when we allowed our daughters to take up their places at the Royal Ballet School. As

I face up to our responsibilities as parents, I understand that it is not enough to be 'well-intentioned'. Like so many risks in life, not everyone suffers; it is not universally bad for every child, but boarding school can ruin not just a childhood but their adult lives as well. I would urge every parent at the very least, to do some research so they are cognisant of the potential harms of boarding before making a decision over their child's schooling.

Recently I have been on several weekends with boarding school survivors where together we have been led by experienced therapists in healing exercises and rituals. I was astonished to also meet my adolescent self who had been hiding within, stuck in her anger, resentment and bitterness over the rejection and abandonment of the past. Through the group activities, I was able to let go of so many feelings which had come to the fore when triggered by difficult events which reminded her of what she had been through.

Without the support and love of Peter by my side, I may never have recovered from the breakdowns during my adult life. Yet, I have been forced to do most of it on my own. In the last seven years, finally I have been able to make significant progress with the support of therapists and others who understood the damaged child within. At last, I have learned that rather than recycle my 'list of failures', the time has come to tear it up and consign it to the bin. I have needed to understand that loving and forgiving my adult self as well as the child and adolescent 'Emily' is the only way that I can really help other people. This is not to say that I was unwilling to take responsibility for the mistakes I have made but rather it becomes an opportunity for reflection and re-evaluation. In the past, I judged myself every time I 'fell over', now I can credit myself for getting back up and for the efforts I have made to carry on.

\* \* \*

*Culture change is never easy. But as activists, peers, ex-boarders or survivors with lived experience, we are not alone and there is so much we can learn from one another. Perhaps together we can shorten the journey to a meaningful life, if not to full recovery. Have you thought about ways of connecting with others, or ways of telling your story?*

# CHAPTER 35

# Liberation

Mid-pandemic, I resumed contact with Gina and together we began the process of reinterpreting Emily's life history.

## CHILD

I accepted that Emily was never a 'bad' child, but she was vulnerable and became highly susceptible to coercion. This first manifested as an eight-year-old, when she tried to gain her parents' attention by making up a story. Instead of feeling loved and comforted, this little girl became utterly terrified, convinced that she was wicked and would be sent to prison. Such an erroneous belief during Emily's time of great need became the foundation stone which led to a lifelong conviction that she deserved to be punished. Within the year, Emily was sent away to boarding school, where she felt abandoned. She was subsequently deprived of the emotional care and attention she needed during her turbulent experience as an adolescent. Here, she learnt a whole raft of dysfunctional coping mechanisms.

Emily suffered very real psychological injury as a child, which contributed to her breakdown in 1994. At this point an understandable emotional crisis resulted from the convergence of the unique set of circumstances. It was the car crash of different strands of tension, stress, and experiences, triggered by memories of boarding school. The validity and context of Emily's life, past and present, were not given sufficient merit by the healthcare professionals with whom she made contact. Perhaps the outcome could have been wildly different if she hadn't been sucked into the healthcare system which medicalised her feelings.

## SUSCEPTIBILITY

For years, even as an adult, she sought love and acceptance in all the wrong places, falling under the influence of a fundamentalist version of Christianity, through branches of the charismatic, evangelical church. As a young doctor, she worked in a profession which was dominated by an authoritarian, patriarchal hierarchy. Bullying was rife and junior doctors rarely questioned their superiors.

There was a considerable imbalance of power and Emily was already highly susceptible to coercion when she was further disempowered by dint of her status as a vulnerable psychiatric patient. She had little agency, while subjected to the opinion of consultant psychiatrists and not only believed that they were more expert than she was, but also thought they had her best interests at heart. Emily had no insight into her deference towards male authority figures when she handed over control to her doctors without the benefits of informed consent. She was unable to seriously question either the diagnosis or the treatment that they 'recommended'. This, combined with the knowledge that failure to comply would lead either to detention in hospital and forced treatment for her psychiatric condition under a section of the Mental Health Act, or the revocation of her licence to practise medicine, ensured her compliance.

## BIAS

In 2005, when the psychiatrist told Emily that depression might be recurring, attribution bias went unrecognised. Instead of recognising normal stress, she was re-prescribed antidepressants which had never helped in the past. During the following year, when Emily moved and encountered a series of difficult circumstances, her lifelong, habitual, and dysfunctional coping mechanisms did not do her any favours. She was diagnosed with a relapse of major depression.

Despite her recovery, psychiatrists persistently predicted future recurrences of depression, coupled with warnings that failure to comply with treatment would inevitably lead to another serious episode. Emily was terrified by the prospect of further hospital admissions and a repeat of her nightmarish experiences. Furthermore, none of the treatment Emily received from NHS psychiatric services adequately dealt with the root causes of her psychological distress. I remain curious why it was, that not one person in mental health services managed to figure out the root cause of my problems and how long it took for me to find the relevant material for myself. In summary, it had been a disastrous and costly exercise not just for the NHS but for Emily and her family as well.

I never chose to be a victim to my circumstances, but now I could see the benefits that can be gained from growing through adversity. It takes strength and courage to survive but when cherished, it can become a tremendous opportunity to help others. I cannot deny the reality of what I suffered, nor the pain and the torment, which was so horrendous that there was a time when I didn't want to carry on living. But here I am, free at last from the shackles of psychiatry, free from the shackles of evangelicalism and free from the shackles placed on a young child sent away to boarding school.

Recovery means different things to different people but unlike beauty, which is in the eye of the beholder, it should be defined by the person who feels they are better. I was a hopeless case defined by a psychiatric diagnostic label, one that robbed me of hope for recovery and hope for the future. There are no guarantees and I do not know whether I will experience severe emotional distress again. Only life will tell. But I know this, where there is life, hope for recovery remains.

\* \* \*

*I hope you have been injected with hope now that the book comes to an end. Please pass it on to someone else if it has been helpful to you. Best wishes for your future recovery journey.*

# Postscript Challenge

## BRANDING

While receiving a psychiatric diagnosis may provide transient relief enabling an individual to name what they are going through or give them access to much-needed help, it is important for the public to be aware of the 'branding' of such diagnoses. Whole industries have grown up around the medicalisation of distress, whether in the form of self-help books, courses, expensive evaluations or the appropriation of psychiatric diagnoses to justify the marketing and prescription of psychotropic drugs. As individuals, we have been led to believe that certain patterns of emotional experience is 'illness' when there is no proof of any abnormality. This so-called 'epidemic' of mental health problems, actually evidences that as human beings we share similarities in the way we respond to the stress of everyday living. If we go to the doctor suffering pain or distress to the extent that we are offered drug treatment for what is deemed a psychiatric condition, then patients must not be under any illusions.

While psychiatric drugs may help alleviate the intensity of feelings *for some people* in the short-term, they are not a cure. Furthermore, it must never be forgotten that these drugs can cause serious and sometimes dangerous adverse effects in an unpredictable manner, as well as horrendous and long-lasting withdrawal symptoms. It is also important for doctors to understand that because their patients are feeling desperate when they seek help, they are more susceptible and may agree to anything which holds the possibility of alleviating their symptoms.

These individuals in particular require adequate support and care as well as time before they can make an informed decision. It is important for all patients everywhere to be empowered; they need to know enough about the truth to weigh up the evidence, rather than be dictated to by those who are deemed to be the experts. Unfortunately, it is easy to be swamped by what is available on the internet and decision-making is not easy when the right information is withheld, or false information is freely available.

## RESTORATIVE JUSTICE

In psychiatry, patients are particularly vulnerable, and all should be given the possibility of independent advocacy, particularly if they are finding it difficult to reach their own conclusions.

We must also be mindful that a psychiatric patient who complains that something is wrong with the system or the treatment they receive is in a double bind. Our words are so easily dismissed as someone who is 'not of sound mind'. Our emotional distress and torment makes it near impossible for us to prove our allegations even after we recover. The courts will not allow us to speak once a significant time has passed, yet it can take decades or more to get to a place where we are in a fit state to understand what happened. Even family and friends are less likely to believe what a psychiatric patient says when their words are pitted against the denials from staff whose actions go unobserved behind the closed doors of a locked ward. Nobody wants to believe a mental patient. It takes undercover reporting such as the recent BBC *Panorama* programme[1] to bring the abuses on locked psychiatric wards to light. This is a travesty.

## PEER SUPPORT

Thankfully, peer support groups have arisen amongst the ever-increasing population of people who have spent years on antidepressants and/or antipsychotics (as well as opiates, benzodiazepines and gabapentinoids.) These groups of experienced patients have been invaluable in drawing the medical profession's attention to the symptoms which occur when people are trying to get off their medication. They have been the driving force behind the current recognition that psychotropic drugs can be very harmful, and if their use cannot be avoided, then they should be used for as short a time as possible. Ideally, the plan to withdraw should be made at the time of the first prescription.

## RETHINK

Modern medicine has benefited greatly from scientific discovery and with additional knowledge, many lives have been saved. But however unwittingly, some attempts to treat disease have done great harm. There is still so much that doctors do not know and so many disease processes that at best can only be modified rather than cured. The medical profession has subsumed its power and are held to be the authorities on health and well-being, and so it is all the more necessary that we are utterly transparent

---

1    BBC 1 *Panorama: Undercover Hospital Patients at Risk*, September 2022

and admit our failings. We must make sure, particularly in psychiatry that we do not deceive patients or coerce patients into accepting advice or treatment. Psychiatrists are powerful, they can legally insist that patients are treated against their will. This should be rare and a last resort. It is paramount that we learn from other nations how to make this an absolute exception to usual practice.

## CHALLENGE TO GOVERNMENT

While the government looks at the deficit as a result of coronavirus, and the future needs of the NHS, it is not a moment too soon to be wise about where money is spent. Trying to fix people within the dominant biomedical psychiatric paradigm based on pseudoscience, is as pointless as giving cigarettes to the troops during wartime or giving alcoholic drinks to hospitalised patients instead of clean water. We look back at those errors with incredulity – how much more will future generations view our vain attempts to medicalise societal problems?

## CHALLENGE TO PSYCHIATRY

I am issuing a challenge particularly to doctors who have trained in psychiatry. I hope they can muster enough courage to take a good hard look at what has been propagated as truth by their profession. With the exception of the dementias and a few rare genetic conditions, there are no confirmatory tests as there are for physical diagnoses. Will they admit that 'psychiatric diagnoses' as listed in the DSM and ICD, like those used in common parlance like depression, anxiety, schizophrenia, OCD, autism and ADHD are nothing other than labels which describe patterns or groups of similar experiences? Will they be brave enough to listen to the many patients who have been harmed, and those who have failed to benefit from their services? Will they speak out about the societal harms which are at the root of so much of their patients' suffering? Will they admit that neither drugs nor ECT can undo the patients' traumatic experiences? Will they be brave enough to modify their prescribing and reduce the possibility of long-term harm from the effects of psychotropic drugs? Holistic and personalised care should be the bedrock of any health service and we must never forget that each and every patient has to be seen in the context of the whole of their lives. It may seem an impossible goal, in today's busy and challenging environments, but all of us would do well to learn to trust people over processes and that means relearning the art of listening.

## CHALLENGE TO SOCIETY

I am also issuing a challenge to a society where there is tacit approval of children being taking away from their homes and placed in institutional care, known as boarding schools, whether paid for by the state or by wealthy middle-class parents. Of course, there may be times when children have to be removed from cruelty or other forms of abuse in their homes, but this should be extremely unusual, and every effort made to find alternatives where they receive love, acceptance, and support from appropriately vetted and trained adults. While boarding schools continue to be regarded as a privilege, it is an indictment on our society, and we will continue to pay an extremely high cost.

# Bibliography and Further Reading

1. Beard, Richard Sad Little Men, Vintage, London, 2022
2. Beddoe, Rebekah Dying for a Cure, Hammersmith Press, London 2009
3. Bentall, Richard P Doctoring the Mind: Why psychiatric treatments fail, Penguin, London, 2010
4. Bentall, Richard P Madness Explained: Psychosis and Human Nature, Penguin, London, 2004
5. Blackford Newman, Katinka The Pill That Steals Lives, John Blake, London, 2016
6. Boyle, Mary & Johnstone, Lucy A Straight Talking Introduction to the Power Threat Meaning Framework, PCCS Books, Monmouth, 2020
7. Davies, James Sedated: How Modern Capitalism Created Our Mental Health Crisis, Atlantic Books, London, 2022
8. Davies, James Cracked: Why Psychiatry is Doing More Harm Than Good, Icon Books, London, 2014
9. Duffell, Nick The Making of Them: The British attitude to Children and the boarding school system, Lone Arrow Press, London, 2000
10. Gøtzsche, Peter C Survival in an Overmedicated World: Look Up the Evidence Yourself, People's Press, 2019

11. Hari, Johann Lost Connections: Why you're depressed and how to find hope, Bloomsbury, London, 2018

12. Hari, Johann Stolen Focus: Why You Can't Pay Attention, Bloomsbury, London, 2022

13. Middleton, Hugh Psychiatry Reconsidered: From Medical Treatment to Supportive Understanding, Palgrave MacMillan, London, 2015

14. Moncrieff, Joanna A Straight talking Introduction to Psychiatric Drugs, PCCS Books, Monmouth, 2009

15. Russo, Jasna & Sweeney, Angela (edited by) Searching for a Rose Garden, PCCS Books, Monmouth, 2016

16. Schaverien, Joy Boarding School Syndrome, Routledge, Abingdon, 2015

17. Stibbe, Mark Home at Last: Freedom from Boarding School Pain, Malcolm Down Publishing, 2016

18. Timimi, Sami Insane Medicine, 2020

19. Van der Kolk, Bessel The Body Keeps the Score: Brain, Mind and Body in the Healing of Trauma, Penguin, New York, 2015

20. Watson, Jo Drop the Disorder: challenging the culture of psychiatric diagnosis, PCCS Books, Monmouth, 2016

21. Whitaker, Robert Anatomy of an Epidemic, Crown, New York, 2011

22. Whitaker, Robert Mad In America, Basic Books, New York, 2019

23. Wield, Cathy Life After Darkness; a doctor's journey through severe depression, CRC press, Oxford, 2006

24. Wield, Cathy A Thorn In My Mind: mental illness, stigma and the church, Instant Apostle, Watford, 2012

25. Young, Terence Death by Prescription, Key Porter Books, Toronto, 2009

# Appendix

**www.adisorder4everyone.com** A Disorder For Everyone (AD4E) hosts events that challenge the dominant diagnostic culture in 'mental health' and brings together people who want change in the understanding and response to emotional distress.

**www.antidepressantrisks.org** Standing up for a safer world. A team of experts with the goal of helping people understand the risks of taking antidepressants.

**www.bacp.co.uk/about-us/protecting-the-public/bacp-register** Register of counsellors and psychotherapists.

**www.boardingschoolsurvivors.co.uk** Therapeutic help for those affected by boarding.

**www.bss-support.org.uk** Help for boarding school survivors to understand and recover from their boarding experience

**www.doi.org/10.1016/j.euroneuro.2021.10.001** Very important book: How to reduce and stop psychiatric medication by Mark Horowitz and David Taylor:

**www.gottman.com/blog/research-still-face-experiment** The experiments looking at reactions of babies to mothers who withhold their expressions.

**www.leap4pdd.org/tapering** Articles from Lived and Professional Experience Advisory Panel for Prescribed Drug Dependence.

www.madinamerica.com/ Mad in America serves as a catalyst for rethinking psychiatric care in the United States (and abroad).

www.madintheuk.com Sister site to Mad in America, Mad in the UK's mission is to serve as a catalyst for fundamentally re-thinking theory and practice in the field of mental health in the UK, and promoting positive change.

www.mind.org.uk/information-support/guides-to-support-and-services/advocacy/types-of-advocacy Provision of advocacy for mental health.

www.nature.com/articles/s41380-022-01661-0 Professor Joanna Moncrieff and other authors -The serotonin theory of depression: a systematic umbrella review of the evidence

www.rcpsych.ac.uk/mental-health/treatments-and-wellbeing/stopping-antidepressants Royal College of Psychiatry advice on stopping antidepressants.

www.rethink.org/advice-and-information/rights-restrictions/rights-and-restrictions/advocacy-for-mental-health Rethink advocacy services and information.

www.seenheard.org.uk Supporting the emotional wellbeing of past and present pupils of boarding & independent day schools, and their families.

www.survivingantidepressants.org Helpful information from those with lived experience of taking antidepressants & withdrawal.

www.space.org.uk/2020/10/06/letter-to-a-mental-health-patient-from-a-psychiatrist-turned-humble Helpful letter as part of Queen Mary University conversations.

www.withdrawal.theinnercompass.org The Withdrawal Project: helpful advice from those with lived experience of withdrawing from psychiatric drugs

# Drugs Emily was prescribed

## ANTIDEPRESSANTS

- Selective serotonin reuptake inhibitors (SSRIs)
  Fluoxetine
  Citalopram
  Paroxetine
  Sertraline

- Tricyclic antidepressants (TCAs)
  Amitriptyline
  Lofepramine
  Dothiepin/ Dosulepin
  Imipramine
  Clomipramine

- Serotonin-noradrenalin reuptake inhibitors (SNRI)
  Venlafaxine

- Serotonin antagonists and reuptake inhibitors (SARI)
  Trazodone

- Monoamine oxidase inhibitors (MAOI)
  Phenelzine

- Noradrenalin and specific serotonergic antidepressants (NASSA)
  Mirtazapine
  Reboxetine

## ANTI-PSYCHOTICS

- Old type
  Chlorpromazine
  Clopixol
  Droperidol
  Flupentixol
  Thioridazine

- Atypicals
  Olanzapine
  Risperidone
  Quetiapine

- Depot (injectable) anti-psychotics
  Depot depixol

## 'MOOD STABILISERS'

  Lithium
  Sodium Valproate

## OTHER DRUGS SPECIFICALLY USED AS 'ADJUNCTIVE THERAPY' TO TREAT INTRACTABLE DEPRESSION

Tryptophan
Ketoconazole
Triiodothyronine

## BENZODIAZEPINES AND Z-DRUGS

Clonazepam
Diazepam
Lorazepam
Nitrazepam
Temazepam
Zolpidem
Zopiclone

## PSYCHOACTIVE DRUGS USED TO COUNTERACT SIDE EFFECTS

Domperidone
Metoclopramide
Procyclidine

## ADDITIONAL DRUGS PRESCRIBED SOLELY TO TREAT THE ADVERSE EFFECTS

Gabapentin
Levothyroxine
Lignocaine cream
Nifedipine

# Glossary

A&E: Accident & Emergency

ADHD: Attention Deficit & Hypersensitivity Disorder
AIS: Advanced Interventions Service – for treating psychiatric patients in Dundee

BACP: British Association for Counselling and Psychotherapy

CBASP: Cognitive Behavioural Analysis System of Psychotherapy

CBT: Cognitive Behavioural Therapy

CSF: Cerebral Spinal Fluid

CT: Computerised tomography ( a 'scan')
DOP: Department of Psychiatry – at Southampton Royal South Hants Hospital

ECFMG: Educational Commission for Foreign Medical Graduates

ECT: Electroconvulsive Therapy
EMDR: Eye Movement Desensitisation and Reprocessing – psychotherapy that helps people process and recover from past trauma using side to side eye movements

ERAS: Enhanced Recovery After Surgery
FMG: Foreign Medical Graduate (in USA)

GCSE: – exams taken in British schools at age sixteen

GP: General Practitioner – primary care doctor

HFASS: House for All Sinners and Saints – church in Denver

HCA: Healthcare Assistant

HH: Holy Helpers

HR: Human Resources

MAOI: Monoamine Oxidase Inhibitor – type of antidepressant

MRI: Magnetic Resonance Imaging
NMD: Neurosurgery for Mental Disorder (also known as psychosurgery)

Obs: Constant observations by nurses on wards

OCD: Obsessive-Compulsive Disorder

PTSD: Post Traumatic Stress Disorder

SHO: Senior House Officer – junior doctor after first year

SpR: Specialist Registrar – junior doctor training in speciality training

SR: Senior Registrar – junior doctor in last year of speciality training
USMLE: United States Medical Licensing Examination

# Acknowledgments

I would like to extend my heartfelt gratitude to the following people for their encouragement and practical help which has helped shape Unshackled Mind – my husband Phil, Mike Hasko, Dr Sami Timimi, Sally Paul, Sue Smith, Dr Duncan Double, James Fielding, Chris Thomas, Hayley Allan and Professor Joanna Moncrieff. There are too many others to name including the friends who voted on the best title for the book. What I will say is without your friendship and support, I would not have been able to fulfil my commitment to re-write the story of my life.